DEDICATION

This book is dedicated to every single dieter around the world who has followed all "the rules" only to end up heavier and more frustrated than before they started. May this book be a fresh perspective and serve as a catalyst for you to unlock the hidden keys to that stubborn weight loss once and for all.

TABLE OF CONTENTS

WHY AM I
STILL FAT?

The Hidden Keys
to Unlocking That
Stubborn Weight Loss

BY DIETITIAN CASSIE, RD, LD

Why Am I Still Fat?
The Hidden Keys To Unlocking That Stubborn Weight Loss

"*Why Am I Still Fat?* is a refreshing explanation for why so many people have failed at dieting, and a step-by-step program outlining how to work through each key to your weight loss success."

>   – Kevin Gianni, author of *Kale and Coffee: A Renegade's Approach to Health, Happiness and Longevity*

"Honest from the start, Dietitian Cassie has written a book that presents the truth through enlightening stories and entertaining writing! If you're stuck in your health and weight-loss journey, *Why Am I Still Fat?* is a book you need!"

>   – Sam Feltham, Director of the Public Health Collaboration, www.phcuk.org

"Dietitian Cassie breaks the rules when it comes to conventional diet advice with a science-based approach that's provided success for her thousands of clients.

Her book has the insider info you won't find anywhere else."

>   – Caitlin Weeks, NC, author of *Mediterranean Paleo Cooking* and www.grassfedgirl.com

PART 3
Key Maximizers: Remember These S's for Fewer "Lbs" 97

PART 4
Amplify Your Efforts 143

HOW TO READ THIS BOOK

While you may be tempted to skip ahead to chapters with headings that resonate the most with you, I encourage you to hang tight with me through each chapter. As you'll soon learn, everything is connected, and sometimes it takes finding the first key to your weight loss in order to discover the next one.

While this book is rather comprehensive in nature, I've also created numerous guides specifically designed to help you with each component. They are an excellent tool to keep on hand for your reference, and also serve as companions to this book.

You can download all of those guides right now at dietitiancassie.com/bonus so that you have them to refer to as you work through each chapter of this book.

I'm so very excited for you to discover the keys within the pages of this book! I know how frustrating the weight loss journey can be, especially when you don't have all the information. One missing piece can mean no weight loss at all, or even a ton of added pounds. So, congratulations on taking this journey and making it this far! Choosing yourself isn't always an easy decision, but it's always a worthwhile one. I'm honored to be your guide and to show you the steps you need to take in order to finally reach that weight loss finish line. Without further ado, let's get started!

PROLOGUE

HAPPY TEARS

She burst into tears, trembling in that comfy brown chair in my office. "This is the first time in my life that I feel understood!"

Before seeing me, she had tried "every diet on the planet," yet the pounds continued to creep on.

"I watch what I eat closer than anyone I know. I measure my portions. I count every calorie, and I exercise almost every day of the week. I never indulge in dessert, and I don't drink alcohol."

She thought something was wrong with her. She had been two clicks away from purchasing yet another detox in an attempt to shed the pounds. She hesitated because she had tried several of those before. She knew the cycle. Get excited. Start the program. Feel the starvation. Eat again. Watch the pounds pack back on.

That's when she saw me on her local television station. She recognized my name from various articles from the Huffington

Post, TIME, Cosmopolitan, SHAPE, and SELF. That day, I was busting the calorie myth, and I encouraged viewers to eat more fat to shed pounds. She liked the sound of that! So, instead of clicking to buy another detox program, she clicked over to my site and scheduled her first appointment.

As we talked, she was surprised to hear my own frustrating journey to lose weight. "You seem so put together—I never would have thought you'd struggled with your weight or food before, too."

"I did, indeed. There was a time not so long ago when I was just as confused and maybe even more frustrated than you are right now. And I was a dietitian even then! If dietitians are confused when it comes to weight loss, then what chance does everyone else have?"

I went on to tell her my story. I told her how my wakeup moment was the night I ate the entire container of my roommate's frosted sugar cookies. At first, I thought I'd just sneak one…or two, and before I knew it, all twelve were gone. It's the kind of embarrassment you never forget. I felt so ashamed when I had to fess up to her. It feels weird to say, but I honestly felt like I couldn't control myself. It didn't even feel like a choice. I *had* to eat them, simply because they were *there*. To make matters worse, I was in school to be a Registered Dietitian! I felt like a fraud—like I was living two lives. I was acing all of my classes, but behind closed doors, I was failing.

To tell the truth, those cookies weren't my only overindulgence. There were hundreds of other moments just like it. Midnight cookie dough runs. Rearranging my schedule to swing by the dessert table between classes. Intentionally buying "Halloween candy" in August. Hitting up McDonald's for Shamrock Shakes in March. Downing Pumpkin Spice Lattes at Starbucks in September. Buying jugs of Eggnog right after Thanksgiving. I consumed them all like they were going out of style—because they were! With each "new" season, I continued to knowingly fall for every marketing trick in the book, but I couldn't stop myself.

I can't count the number of times I tried to get a fresh start, or do a sugar detox, only to wind up in the same place in a matter of days. Every time I would be a little more angry at myself for being too weak to control it—breaking my own promises and not being able to stick to my decisions. Maybe there was just something wrong with me.

Years later, I realized I had a sugar addiction. Most people don't know or believe it, but sugar has the same effect on the brain as cocaine. It triggers the same reward centers. Sugar sensitivity is real. And for many people, it's debilitating.

I was an addict.

Ironically, the eating regimen I was learning in dietitian school at the time—the low-fat, low-calorie diet—added fuel to the fire. It took me on a blood sugar roller coaster ride that brought me to the unhealthiest point of my life. But then something happened that pushed me over the edge.

It was my last year of dietitian school when I got the call. My father had to have unexpected, major heart surgery. For as long as I could remember, he was the picture of health, following all "the rules," exercising regularly and eating low-calorie and low-fat, and yet he ended up in the hospital. Something didn't add up. After surgery, his doctors and dietitians adamantly told him to maintain his low-calorie, low-fat diet.

That's when I got angry. "This diet is what landed him here on your operating table!" That's when I was determined to figure it out on my own. I had to become my own advocate, so I could be my dad's advocate, too.

I looked at all of the scientific research and studies, and I was astonished by the conclusions. I had to do the exact *opposite* of practically everything I'd been learning in school! What I'd been learning wasn't research-based and wasn't even working. They said to avoid egg yolks, but then I found that eggs are good for the heart. They said to use margarine, but then I found that butter is healthier than a substance made in a lab. They said to drink soy milk, but then I found that soy can disrupt hormonal balance. They said to load up on bread and pasta, but these carbs fuel sugar addiction!

Soon after, I quit the low-fat and low-cal dieting. I started eating eggs for breakfast, adding butter to my veggies, and avocado to my smoothies. I ate more fat and more food in general. Amazingly, I stopped being consumed with thoughts of sugar. Gone were the days without energy. My brain had never felt more clear and powerful. I lost the "Freshman Fifteen" (twenty if we're being honest) effortlessly.

Fast forward to today: I'm in the best shape of my life. I never thought this was possible! For so long, I had believed that a sugar addiction was just part of my identity, my genetics…me. That was a lie.

It's no wonder our country is getting fatter and sicker. There's too much misinformation out there based on outdated research contained in dusty old textbooks. We've spent decades following low-calorie, low-fat diets while busting our butts at the gym and feeling like failures. After all this, we're still not losing weight.

That's why I've made it my personal mission to share the power of real food with as many people just like you as I possibly can. That's what *Why Am I Still Fat?* is all about.

Our thousands of clients at *Healthy Simple Life*—the company I founded to spread health and nutrition facts—are seeing the results they've been looking for thanks to our up-to-date science-based program. We see tears of joy streaming from their eyes when they overcome challenges they never thought they could overcome. This book is the next step towards reaching even more people with the incredible power of real food.

Today, I can confidently say that I have control over my sugar addiction—and I want you to have that control over the hurdles in your life, too. I bet your story is similar to mine: you've struggled with something like a sugar addiction, a fast food addiction, or perhaps weight loss for far too long, and you just can't get to the bottom of it no matter how many diets you try or how many healthcare professionals you see. I'm excited to tell you that you're in the right place!

Throughout my journey, I've come to learn that it's not just about food. It's not just about exercise either. Those are the two areas I studied in school—and yet weight loss is about so much more than that. The strategies we've developed at *Healthy Simple Life* really work, and our clients' results are the best possible proof of that.

Remember the client with the happy tears? She went through exactly what is outlined in this book. She didn't mind that this wasn't just another "quick fix" when she saw that the weight she had lost was *staying off*. She felt like a new person, and to this day, she knows she can keep that fabulous feeling for the rest of her life. That's because we focused on healing from the inside out and addressed some key factors that she never considered before. Our plan isn't a band-aid—it's a solution.

So, this isn't your typical weight loss book. I'm not going to tell you to count your calories, eat 100-calorie packs of low-fat cookies, and use a margarine spread instead of butter to lose weight. In fact, I'm going to tell you to do just the opposite. This book is a compilation of the (sometimes surprising) factors that come into play when it comes to weight loss.

Don't be alarmed, but this may be the first time you hear a dietitian telling you to eat more fat...and that it's good for your heart. Now, it's completely natural to be skeptical. After all, we've been brainwashed to believe fat is our enemy since the 70's.

In this book, I'm going to challenge a lot of what you may know as "truth." The reason for that is because these supposed "truths" never worked for me, haven't worked for our clients, and frankly, a lot of them conflict with what the research studies are actually reporting. More often than not, in the case of nutrition, weight loss wisdom from food manufacturers, the media, and maybe even your practitioner, simply isn't in line with scientific evidence. I know you're here because the same health claims that didn't work for me aren't working for you either. So, I invite you to keep an open mind as you work through the chapters of this book.

If you've been on "every diet on the planet" and still can't figure out why you're not losing weight, then you are exactly where you are supposed to be; this is the book for you. While I will be covering the importance of the food you're eating, I very well might be the first dietitian to tell you that as important as nutrition is, it's not all about food.

It is time to abandon calorie counting and low-fat diets. We've been misled and manipulated—and not given the full story. I'm going to ask you to forget just about everything you thought you knew about weight loss and help you open your mind to a new way of living. There are several non-dietary reasons why you might not be losing weight. In the following chapters, I'll reveal to you the hidden keys I've found that have unlocked that stubborn weight loss for thousands of our clients. Now it's your turn.

PART 1

FOOD:
STOP RESTRICTING,
START EATING

CHAPTER ONE

HORMONES, NOT CALORIES –
THE LIE YOU'VE BEEN FED

A Flawed Theory

On one of my first days on the job working as a dietitian, I had a patient come in with a feeding tube. A feeding tube is a device used to provide nutrition to people who cannot eat orally. This patient was receiving all of his nutrition through the tube, which means I could control every last calorie he was taking in. I knew without a doubt he wasn't "cheating" because this was his only source of nutrition and sadly, he couldn't eat orally even if he wanted to. The day I first met with him, he was on an 800 calorie per day diet. Ironically, he had gained 10 pounds since the last time he'd seen a dietitian, just months prior. As I read through the notes the previous dietitian had documented, I noticed a trend happening—as his calories were reduced (from 1800 to 1500 to 1200 to 1000 to now currently 800…) his weight went up. But, why? Thankfully, I wasn't stumped for long. I realized that it was due to a lot of the non-caloric, non-food factors that I outline in the coming chapters of this book. Not about calories. If it were all about calories, he would have, without a doubt, been losing weight as his daily calorie intake decreased. That's how it was supposed to work anyway…right? Well, not quite.

I know you've been told over and over to count your calories and make sure you're burning more than you're taking in. If you're not, then you won't lose weight. If you are, and you're still not losing weight, then you're too indulgent, don't have enough willpower, or there's something wrong with you.

Of course, this advice is shameful, flat out false, and heartbreaking. There are several more factors that play a role in how your metabolism functions and whether you're losing or gaining weight—beyond "calories in and calories out." True weight loss that stays off is never about deprivation.

Time and time again, clients have come to me who have been counting calories to a "T", yet, like my patient on the feeding tube, they can't seem to lose weight. They even sometimes gain weight in the process. Or they lose weight and then gain it all back when they finally eat again (because we can't starve ourselves forever!). Maybe this is starting to sound a little too familiar to you. Let me explain why this happens.

Your body is extremely complex. Trying to oversimplify by tracking a single substance, like a calorie, is ineffective and frankly, degrading. Counting calories leaves you feeling deprived, dissatisfied, and hungry and eventually, right back where you started (or worse). Not only do you feel lethargic and empty as you restrict your body of what it needs (energy in the form of calories), but any weight you do lose ends up coming back anyway once you start eating again. It's a lose-lose situation. Not only do you not attain the desired result, but you also feel awful in the process and horrible about yourself! To make matters worse, you end up slowing down your metabolism—actually damaging it, which makes your next attempt at shedding pounds even more difficult. Calorie counting isn't just ineffective; it sets you up for yo-yo weight loss and gain for years to come. It's a battle you are destined to lose. Can someone please tell me why we are still continuing this madness?!

The Science of Energy

Okay, let's back up: by definition, a calorie is the energy it takes to raise the temperature of one gram of water by one degree Celsius. The important takeaway from this definition is the word *energy*. Calories are energy that fuel our bodies and help them run; just like gasoline fuels our cars. You wouldn't expect your car to run better if you take away the gas, so why would you expect your body to work better when you deprive it of calories? That's why restricting calories for weight loss doesn't make any sense. When you deprive your body of the energy it needs, it fights back and actually conserves its own energy by slowing down your metabolism (or the speed of your car, in our example). That's why when you follow a diet, you feel tired, irritable, hungry, have outrageous cravings, frequent headaches, and low energy levels. The opposite is true as well: when you fuel your body with what it needs, it works for you; you are satisfied and lose weight.

So when you think of calories, think of energy. Do the same when you hear the word *metabolism*.

Metabolism is a term I'll continue to use throughout this book. Your metabolism is how efficiently your body is able to convert the things you eat and drink into energy. How much body fat you store and how much you're able to burn is a function of your metabolism. When you provide your body with the right type of calories (which we'll get into in the next section), you fuel your metabolism and keep it revved up, which allows you to lose weight.

So, eat fewer calories and your body burns fewer calories. Eat more and your body burns more. The more you fuel the fire, the more it burns. When it burns, you feel energetic, you can think clearly, and if the other factors we'll discuss soon are in balance, you'll be able to effortlessly shed pounds. This is the opposite of dieting where you feel lethargic, have a foggy brain, and your body fights against you by conserving energy instead of burning it. That's the reason nearly all calorie counters gain the weight back after they lose it.

"Calories in and calories out" is a fundamentally flawed view. One obvious reason is that this theory treats all calories equally, regardless of source, and calories are not created equal. Your body does not metabolize and process all calories in the same way. For instance, some calories consist of chemicals your body doesn't recognize. With the calorie-counting concept, diet soda is equivalent to WATER. Does that make sense? No way! Your body doesn't treat diet soda the same way it treats water! Research repeatedly shows that artificial sweeteners can cause weight gain; they hinder your metabolism since your body doesn't recognize them. We will take a look at that topic more in Chapter Fifteen.

An Introduction to PFC

There are three macronutrient categories that every food falls into: protein, fat, or carbohydrate. While many foods overlap into two or all three categories, for simplicity's sake, it's easiest to designate a food as a protein, fat, or carb based on whichever macro it contains most of. For example, the jar of peanut butter in my fridge says that, per serving, it contains seven grams of protein, seven grams of carbs, and *seventeen* grams of fat. Therefore, it counts as a fat. Pretty easy.

So, why is this helpful? Well, the short answer is that the best way to support your metabolism (and, by extension, your waistline) is to consume all three—proteins, fats and carbohydrates—together, in balance. "PFC Every Three" (short for Protein, Fat, and Carbohydrates) is the term I coined referring to eating a combination of the three macronutrients every few hours.

"I know the goal is to get away from tracking my food, but I can't help it. It's been a habit for so long," MaryAnn said. "So anyway, here's why I'm telling you about my tracking: I realized that I'm eating *double* the amount of calories than when I first saw you last month! I'm *still* losing weight! How is this possible?!"

What MaryAnn experienced isn't uncommon with the clients we work with. When you quit depriving your body and fuel it with the nutrients and energy it needs, magic happens. It has to do with what your body does with your P's, F's and C's.

The three macronutrients, protein, fat and carbohydrates, are processed very differently in the body. We'll dive into each macronutrient deeper, but in general, your proteins are meat, fish and eggs, fats are olive oil, coconut oil, butter, nuts, seeds, olives, avocados and coconut milk, and carbs are fruits and veggies.

Fat, which is the most calorie-dense macronutrient, is essential for long-lasting weight loss. There is a sad irony to how fat is treated in the calorie-counting community. Fat supports metabolism and actually helps us lose weight by buffering the effect of sugar on our bloodstream. Unfortunately, it is the first macronutrient to be eliminated on a calorie-counting diet simply because it has more calories per gram than the other two macronutrients. (Fat has 9 calories per gram, whereas protein and carbohydrates have 4 calories per gram.) Therefore, diets that focus on counting calories are almost always high in carbohydrates and low in fat. It's true that if it were all about counting and restricting calories, it would make sense to eliminate fat to lose weight. However, as you may already know from experience, and as I illustrated with my tube-feeding patient at the beginning of this chapter and now with MaryAnn, it's not just about calories. The amount of calories you burn is controlled by your body and is dependent not just on the quantity, but also the *quality* of the calories you consume.

So, your biology doesn't operate like a single, simple math equation—it's so much more complex. Everything needs to be in balance for you to lose weight. Calorie restriction is not the best way to achieve the long-term weight loss you're looking for because the only thing it takes into account is the amount, not the quality and not the impact it has on your body, hormones, and metabolism.

We need to support our underlying biochemistry and the way our bodies work instead of trying to oversimplify things and assume they will work better if we are restrictive. Cutting calories doesn't address the underlying reason for your lack of weight loss. So, I'm telling you to stop counting calories. It's time to "un-brainwash" yourself from thinking quick fixes are the answer and dig deeper to get to the root cause of your weight concerns.

Hormones, Not Calories

Now, we've established that our ability to metabolize stored fat for energy is not a matter of calories in and calories out, so what is it? Well, it's a matter of *hormonal balance*—one of the common missing pieces of the weight loss puzzle. Your hormones dictate whether your body is burning or storing fat. The first two hormones I'd like to bring to your attention are insulin and glucagon. (Yes, glucagon is a real word—the first time I said "glucagon" on public television, I was asked if it was a *Star Wars* reference.) The hormones insulin and glucagon are in charge of whether or not you are burning or storing fat at any given moment. They can't coexist—it's one or the other.

You can think of insulin as your fat-*storing* hormone and glucagon as your fat-*burning* hormone. You'll want to get cozy and make glucagon your best friend because when glucagon is around, you feel stable, energetic, focused, positive, and best of all, you're burning fat for energy. When insulin is working, the opposite is true: you're a fat-storing machine, packing on the pounds, and feeling lousy in the process.

So how can we keep insulin on the sidelines and glucagon working for us? We should start this conversation by discussing the dreaded *blood sugar roller coaster.*

Whoa, what? Roller coaster?

Hang onto the handrails and let me explain.

Most roller coasters are fun. Your stomach full of butterflies. Anticipating the unknown. The gigantic ups and downs. The delightful dizziness in your head. Most roller coaster rides last two to three minutes. Now, imagine riding a roller coaster all day long…no thanks! While it's fun for a few minutes at an amusement park, when it comes to everyday living, riding the blood sugar roller coaster day in and day out is exhausting. It depletes you of energy, focus, and sets you up for weight gain. It's no way to live. You know you've been for a ride when you're constantly fighting sugar cravings, having trouble focusing, struggling to fall and/or staying asleep, experiencing mood swings, staving off low energy levels and battling with undesired weight gain or having trouble losing weight. Sound familiar?

Here's what's happening: Carbs fuel the roller coaster. Carbohydrates are one of those three macronutrients I mentioned earlier (fat and protein are the other two). When you eat a carbohydrate, regardless of the source (bread, pasta, rice, cookies, candy, soda, and even vegetables and fruits), it turns into sugar the moment it hits your bloodstream. Your blood sugar levels spike, which is alarming to your body, so it triggers your pancreas to quickly secrete that fat-storing hormone I mentioned, insulin. Insulin's job is to unlock the door to your cells, allowing sugar to get into the cell and out of your bloodstream, in turn driving blood sugar levels back down to normal. Ultimately, your body's goal is to bring you down from the top of that roller coaster!

Now, you *can* use that sugar in your bloodstream for energy. If you're active shortly after consuming it, you'll burn it off. The problem is so often we're consuming more sugar than we need, and most of us have desk jobs. We aren't running marathons all day long, and I wouldn't recommend it. When insulin takes that sugar to your cell, the sugar is turned into fat and stored since it's not needed. What happens next? You eat again, which means you don't tap into your fat stores. So you continue to store fat instead of burning it, all day and all night long. I repeat: your body stores that sugar as fat. Carbohydrates, the very foods you've been eating as you've been so focused on eating less fat, have been packing on your pounds. And, the story can get worse.

Resistance to insulin can build up over time, too. The body gradually produces more and more insulin in an attempt to get your cells to work better until they're worn out and don't respond to insulin anymore. Compare this to being in a noisy room—when you walk in, it's loud and you can't hear anything, but after a while you get used to it. When this happens in your body, your pancreas secretes more insulin, and the more that circulates in the body, the harder it becomes to lose weight.

What's happening in your bloodstream? Your blood sugar levels—which were spiked by the carbs—now drop once that sugar is stored in your cells. (Anything that goes up must come down! Thanks a lot, Isaac Newton.) The more carbs you eat in shorter time intervals causes your blood sugar levels to hit their greatest highs and lows. This is what I refer to as the blood sugar roller coaster—the vicious cycle of spikes and drops in blood sugar that happens when following an eating regimen consisting of mostly sugar and carbohydrates (which turn into sugar).

What about glucagon?

Okay, so you understand that eating a lot of carbs and/or sugar take you for a ride on the blood sugar roller coaster, causing your fat-storing hormone, insulin, to do its job and store fat.

Now, what about that magical hormone we want to be best friends with—the one I told you about earlier—glucagon? Here's the key: Glucagon is released by your pancreas to do its job when you're *not* riding the blood sugar roller coaster. It can get to work when your blood sugar levels are nice and stable. Imbalanced blood sugar levels can lead to weight gain, and stable blood sugars are essential for weight loss. Remember, you can't burn fat and store it at the same time. So in order to be in touch with glucagon, we've gotta stay off that roller coaster.

How Do We Stop the Ride and Start Losing Weight?

We get off the roller coaster by having protein and healthy fat with our carbs, every time we eat. "PFC Every Three" is the key to keeping you off the roller coaster because it keeps your blood sugar levels steady.

Here's how it works: You know that carbohydrates, which are the foundation of low-calorie and low-fat diets, cause your fat-storing hormone, insulin, to be released and store fat. Fat and protein, on the other hand, aren't metabolized as sugar. They act as buffers, slowing down the absorption of sugar into your bloodstream and, in turn, help to keep your blood sugar levels stable. Again, when your blood sugars are stable, that wonderful fat-burning hormone, glucagon, is released, which burns stored fat for energy. Get on glucagon's good side by eating more butter and bacon, thus giving glucagon a chance to shine. You come out ahead too, because when your glucagon is rocking and rolling, so are you! You become a fat-burning machine with more energy and a better chance at shedding the pounds.

This, my friend, is why it's not so much about calories as it is about *hormones*! It's time to change the way we think about fat and overcome our unhealthy (and unfounded) fear of it. Remember: carbohydrates and sugar trigger the release of insulin, your fat-storing hormone. Fat doesn't raise your blood sugar levels. Instead, it helps your blood sugar levels stabilize so you can release glucagon, your fat-burning, metabolism-boosting hormone! Healthy fat is a good guy. Of course, protein is important because of its metabolism-boosting effects. Both protein and fat address the satiety factor, meaning they keep you feeling full, too! These are some of the foundations for PFC. There are so many benefits for eating this way. Eating in PFC balance lowers insulin levels and reduces inflammation, another topic we'll dive into shortly, and when this happens, your body works for you, your metabolism runs better, hunger and cravings subside and weight loss happens naturally and automatically—without restriction and deprivation.

Timing Matters

It's not just about what you eat, but also *when* you eat that is important. I've found for both myself and the thousands of clients we've worked with that having a P, F and C every three to four hours—starting within an hour of waking, all the way up until you lay your head on the pillow at night—is the best way to support overall blood sugar balance and weight loss. This could sound overwhelming if you're used to only eating three meals a day, but it doesn't necessarily mean you're eating more food overall. Eating snacks between your meals often results in reduced hunger at mealtimes, so you tend to eat smaller portions. That's because it boosts your metabolism by keeping your blood sugar levels stable. This also lowers your levels of your fat-storing hormone, insulin and supports the release of your fat-burning hormone, glucagon, and in turn, weight loss.

Snacking between your meals is a great preventative measure to stay off the blood sugar roller coaster. When you don't snack, your body learns to live in "starvation mode," and your metabolism slows down as your body adjusts and compensates. Your body then hangs onto extra energy at meals by turning it into fat because it's expecting that it will need that fat in case you don't eat for a while again. Snack on protein, healthy fat, and vegetable and fruit carbohydrates every few hours to keep your metabolism high and to stay in fat-burning mode.

Before we go any further, let's break down each P, F and C category and look at what they are and what they do before tying them all together into your game plan.

CHAPTER TWO

PUNCH UP YOUR PROTEIN

The P in PFC: Protein

When you think of protein, think of meat, fish and eggs. I recommend animal protein because it's the type that turbocharges metabolism the most. It also contains all of the essential amino acids in the perfect proportions, which is important for your skin, hair, heart, and hormones.

Protein is a building block for many of your neurotransmitters (brain chemicals). It can help keep sugar cravings at bay. It also helps your body in its natural detoxification process as it plays a role in eliminating toxins. Protein is important for hormonal balance and, of course, muscle development and growth.

In case I haven't already made it clear: protein is extremely important!

Now, while all of those benefits are great, for the purpose of this book, I'm only going to focus on how protein helps you shed those stubborn pounds—the metabolism-boosting attributes of protein. Protein has the ability to increase the rate of your metabolism every time you eat it. In fact, it can boost your metabolism up to 35 percent for two to three hours after you consume it. Naturally, you can see how it would be beneficial to maintain that boost throughout the day, keeping your metabolism revved up not just at meal time, but at snack time, too.

Speaking of snack time, let's look at a few sources of protein that make for great snacks. My personal favorite protein snacks are hard boiled eggs, dried beef, and chicken sticks. Tuna salad, egg salad, chicken salad, and salmon salad also make for fantastic PFC-balanced snacks. Simply mix the protein source (the canned tuna, chicken, salmon, or chopped up hard boiled eggs) with a couple tablespoons of full fat mayonnaise or olive oil, add chopped grapes and celery, and you have a perfectly balanced PFC snack.

I mentioned eggs as one of the most important protein sources. Now, you may be thinking, "I thought eggs (or at least their yolks) caused heart disease, so how many eggs should I really eat?" Let me be the first to tell you that eggs are good for your heart. Yes, despite what we've been told for five decades, the saturated fat and cholesterol found in egg yolks does not increase your risk for heart disease (as shown in a thoroughly reviewed article that compiled data from decades of research (*Bahl*, 2015), a meta-analysis of data from 72 studies involving 600,000 participants in 18 countries (Chowdhury, 2014),and a meta-analysis of studies in the American Journal of Clinical Nutrition (Siri-Tarino, Sun Q, Hu FB, Krauss RM, 2010)[1]...you get the point). Your heart actually *needs* saturated fat and cholesterol, both of which are heart protective. In fact, it's the foods that have been

---

[1] Siri-Tarino, PW. "Meta-analysis of prospective cohort studies evaluating the ..." 2010. <http://www.ncbi.nlm.nih.gov/pubmed/20071648>

suggested we use in *place* of the eggs that may promote heart disease by creating chronic inflammation in the body. So seriously, eat as many eggs as you like. The information we've heard for years suggesting that eating eggs will cause heart disease is FALSE!

While I encourage eating eggs for heart health, there's one common protein source that I do NOT recommend: soy. Historically, soy has been glamorized as a heart healthy food, but soy protein can alter estrogen levels, decrease thyroid function, and interfere with mineral absorption: all which can halt your weight loss. As I stated earlier, the best kinds of protein are simply from meat, fish, and eggs.

Shake it Up with Protein Powder

Of course, without skipping a beat, whenever conversations shift to protein, protein powders are bound to come up. So, my stance on protein powders is this: they can be really helpful and they can also be really harmful. Personally, I use a protein powder every single day, and I do it for a few reasons. For those times when you're in a pinch with no time to cook, or you don't feel like eating (sick days or post-workout), protein powders are fantastic. I like to make a protein smoothie either for breakfast or a mid-morning snack every day because it's delicious and I jam-pack it with all of my powdered vitamins. You can download that recipe at dietitiancassie.com/smoothie.

However, the problem is not all protein powders are created equal. Most, if not all, protein powders on store shelves are filled with harmful ingredients, including fillers, additives, artificial sweeteners, and all sorts of stuff that stand in the way of your weight loss goal. Not only that, but they can actually cause weight gain! Supplements aren't regulated, and protein powder falls into the supplement category. This means there are no regulatory standards that a protein powder must be subjected to and comply with. Because of this, the protein powders on shelves can be full of junk that's neutral at best and may even be harmful.

The protein powders I personally use and recommend are "pharmaceutical grade" which means they are regulated by a third-party. My favorite whey protein is Ultimate Natural Whey Protein, which is imported from New Zealand, where Recombinant Bovine Growth Hormone (rBGH) is not approved for use—which is a really good thing. In New Zealand, cattle herds graze in pastures year-round—largely avoiding the need for feed supplements such as grain. For that reason, I actually refuse to use other protein powders, and on top of all that, it tastes great too. It has a light vanilla flavor, with no artificial sweeteners or added sugars, and it mixes into liquids and smoothies really well. One of my favorite tricks is mixing it with peanut butter. With protein-packed peanut butter, you can simply spread it onto a banana or some apple slices for a PFC-balanced snack! Check it out at rfvitamins.com/whey.

What about non-whey protein powders? Those can be tricky, too. Again, unless you get pharmaceutical grade, there aren't any standards and they can have a lot of mystery ingredients and harmful junk in them. To help address this issue, I actually put together a guide for you with my best recommendations. You can find this free guide at dietitiancassie.com/protein.

Non-Animal Proteins are Not Complete Proteins

So now that you understand the importance of protein in my PFC-balanced approach to weight loss, you may be wondering if you'll be able to follow this approach if you're a vegetarian or vegan—especially since I told you animal protein is ideal. Well, as a former vegetarian myself, I can speak from experience and say that in those days, I was never fully satisfied after a meal or snack. Even after stuffing my face, I'd have cravings an hour later, and those were almost always for carbs and sugar. Even when trying to pair foods together on my vegetarian eating regimen in an attempt to make up for the lack of animal protein I wasn't consuming, I wasn't satisfied. Looking back, it makes sense as to why not. I didn't realize it at the time, but a vegetarian and vegan way of eating is a high-carb diet. While vegans and vegetarian experts will tell you that you can get plenty of protein from plants, you will have to consume a TON of carbohydrates to get there.

Practically all of the vegetarian protein sources I was diligently consuming to replace my animal protein were actually carbs! For example, when it comes to black beans, a common source of "protein" for vegetarians and vegans alike, a half of a cup of them contains about 20 grams of carbs and only 7 grams of (incomplete) protein. That's nearly three times the amount of carbs as it is protein. Which means, that its PFC category would be carbohydrate—not protein.

When an animal source of protein is replaced by a plant source, you end up getting a lot of extra carbs. On top of that, in order to get an adequate amount of protein at each meal (25 grams is the minimum for most people at meal time), you'd need to consume a cup and a half of those beans. This amounts to 70 grams of carbohydrates, which turns into 17.5 teaspoons of pure sugar the instant it hits your bloodstream! (You can figure this out with any food by dividing the grams of carbohydrate by four to get the teaspoons of sugar it turns into in your body.) Sadly, that's a fast way to hop on that blood sugar roller coaster, and it's exactly why I was dragging along with low energy levels, a foggy brain, sugar cravings and extra weight, all throughout my vegetarian days. I thought I was doing the healthy thing, focusing on plant nutrition, when really, I wouldn't have been much worse off consuming spoonfuls of sugar instead (if that sounds like an exaggeration, don't miss the next chapter!).

To make matters worse, plant sources of protein aren't "complete." They don't contain all of the essential amino acids that an animal protein source would, like an egg or piece of chicken. Proteins are made up of varying combinations of amino acids, which make up the tissues in our body. There are essential amino acids and nonessential amino acids. We have to get the essential ones from the foods we consume. Because animal protein contains all of the essential amino acids in the perfect amounts, it's referred to as a "complete protein," which is ideal. The essential amino acids found in plant substances are not in the ideal proportions and are therefore referred to as "incomplete proteins," which is another reason why getting protein from animal sources like meat, fish and eggs is the best. Many of the vegetarian and vegan carb choices are also high in anti-nutrients. This means they can interfere with the nutrients you're taking in along with them, actually making them worse for you. We'll touch on this more in the carb chapter.

The main takeaway is this: When I couldn't take feeling lousy any longer and I started adding quality animal proteins back into my eating regimen—ditching my soy lattes and veggie burgers—I immediately noticed a surge in my energy levels and, surprisingly, a huge drop in my cravings for carbs and sugar. Hundreds of our clients who have been on a similar journey from a plant-based diet to adding in quality animal sources of protein have experienced much the same results. One of the reasons for this is that when you replace your carb-sources of protein (like beans, rice, veggie burgers and soy products) with animal protein, you're not only taking in better protein, but you're also, by default, reducing your carb intake and thereby eating more PFC-balanced. That means you can stay off the blood sugar rollercoaster that only sets you up for cravings, mood swings, low energy levels and weight gain and with stable blood sugar levels, your energy levels and metabolism boost and pounds drop off.

I'll be upfront and say that vegetarian and vegan diets simply aren't as healthy as ones that contain animal protein, so I don't recommend either of them. That said, I understand that people choose a vegetarian or vegan lifestyle for a lot of reasons, so I completely respect and honor your choice if you decide to not include meat in your diet. You will still reap many of the benefits of a PFC-balanced eating regimen. I've worked with many clients who choose to leave the meat out, and they have still managed to achieve weight loss and other results they were seeking. It's just trickier, and I don't think it's as healthy.

If you're willing to include fish and eggs, it makes things a heck of a lot easier. You can have eggs, fish, or protein powder at all of your meals and snacks, and despite missing out on some of the nutrients that meat contains, you should still be able to get in enough protein to feel great and reach your weight loss goal. I recommend whey protein powder for vegetarians, and if you're a strict vegan, a rice or pea protein powder is better than soy. You can replace the nutrients you'll be missing out on from not eating meat with vitamin B12, iron and a multivitamin supplements, but I would also strongly recommend working with a dietitian coach who can help you fill in these gaps and examine your individualized eating regimen to avoid nutritional deficiencies.

So, let's focus on consuming quality protein to support our weight loss and energy goals!

Embrace: Meat, fish, seafood, eggs, and whey protein powder. Keep it simple and focus on quality. Look for grass-fed, organic meats that are free of added hormones and antibiotics, free-range chicken and turkey and wild game (I love my dad's venison!). This also means you'll be avoiding pesticides and GMOs that are found in the feed of conventionally-raised animals, which aren't good for your metabolism or waistline. Likewise, when it comes to seafood, buy wild-caught fish to ensure you're not consuming heavy loads of chemical residue. Remember, anything your food ate, you're also eating.

Avoid: Food from cows given feed covered in pesticides or farm-raised fish that are fed exclusively genetically modified soy. Processed meats with nitrates or MSG, meat imitation products (tofu, seitan, etc.), soy protein, beans and other carbohydrate sources that are sometimes counted as "meat substitutes" should also be avoided.

Portion: A good rule of thumb is to aim for eating a portion of protein equivalent to the thickness and circumference of the palm of your hand at meals (2-3 eggs, 4-6 oz. of chicken, beef, or fish) and about half that amount for snacks. Your body does not store protein, so you need to make sure you're eating it throughout the day—not too much and not too little. Protein at snack time can be a new concept. Most of us have protein at dinner and are lucky if we have any at lunch or breakfast. Think about incorporating protein *every* time you eat.

CHAPTER THREE

STOP FEARING FAT!

The F in PFC: Fat

Make butter your new best friend. I'm serious.

This is one of the things that brings the most excitement to our clients: permission to eat fat again! Not only is it delicious, but it actually helps you shed pounds! It doesn't hinder weight loss, like we've been wrongly told for too many dreadful years. It's also good for your heart—not bad for it like we've been brainwashed to believe.

I understand that eating fat to lose fat may go against everything you have been taught about weight loss. If you don't want to add fat *to* your body, don't put fat *in* your body. Right? On the surface, it seems to make sense. However, if you've previously eliminated fat from your eating regimen, and you begin reincorporating it, it won't take long for you to notice that you feel more energized. This is because you *need* fat for your metabolism to work properly. (Do you remember what you're supposed to think of when you hear the word metabolism? *Energy!*) Low-fat means low energy, more hunger, and more cravings. Consider the effect different foods have on your mind and body.

Do you feel satisfied when you eat "lite" products? Can you stop after eating a half cup of "low-fat" ice cream? What about "fat-free" yogurt? Fat contributes to satiety, so when you have fat with your meals and snacks, you are less likely to overeat. Compare snacking on nuts and berries to having a "100 calorie" pack of cookies. It's hardly a comparison: the fat in the nuts helps you feel satisfied, whereas the carbohydrates in the cookies, which turn into sugar the instant they hit your bloodstream, leave you craving more. It goes back to the spikes and crashes of riding the blood sugar roller coaster. Fat keeps you stable and in control, and carbs and sugar make you lose your mind with frequent ups and downs.

In spite of all this, ever since the 1970s, we've been obsessed with low-fat foods. Everyone from food marketers to trusted professionals have successfully convinced us to believe that fat is the enemy. To this day, the media still supports this message through its marketing of "low-fat," "lite," "fat-free," and the one I love to hate the most, "skinny" products. While times are slowly changing, we are still being told from a variety of angles that skimping on fat will help with weight loss. Here's the kicker—this fat-phobia was actually never based on any scientific reason! Let's ask ourselves, how has that been working for us? Has the dramatic reduction of fat in our diets really helped us become healthier and less fat? Or is it possible that fat might not really be making us fat? Ever since this avoid-fat-at-all-costs trend began, the United States and many other nations have been packing on more and more pounds, which has lead to the greatest obesity epidemic in world history. Obesity skyrocketed as our fat intake went down. It is time to change the way we think about fat and overcome our unhealthy fear of it.

The Truth About Fat

Fat supports brain function, keeps us full, and acts as a buffer for carbohydrates by slowing down their assimilation into our bloodstream. Every cell in our body relies on fat because our cell membranes are *made* from it. It plays a central role in our nervous system, brain function, skin integrity and mineral absorption, and it has healing and immunity response properties. What you probably care about most is that it supports metabolism! Whew, no wonder it's important!

Fat keeps us full and satiated. When you consume it, a chemical called cholecystokinin is released and sends a signal to your brain, telling it that you're full, so your brain then turns off your appetite. Fat wards off cravings, aids in healthy hormone production, and boosts healing during inflammatory processes. Fat helps lower your risk for diabetes, heart disease, and obesity. Did you know that over sixty percent of your brain is made of fat? This is why your brain doesn't work very well when you're on a low-fat diet; you're depriving your brain of the fat it needs for basic functioning. We NEED healthy fat.

It's time we, as a society, dispel the myth that consuming fat is what makes us fat and begin to embrace the healthy fats that calorie-counting diets won't let us near. The reality is the right types of fat support weight loss, while we should be blaming the processed carbohydrates that are converted to sugar and then stored as fat for our weight gain. Fat acts as a buffer, slowing down the absorption of sugar into your bloodstream, resulting in less stored fat...because fat doesn't turn into fat, sugar does!

Now, I think we can all agree that flavor is highly prioritized in our culture. If something doesn't taste good, we generally avoid it. Common sense, right? Well, because fat is a major source of flavor, if it's removed from our food, something else has to be added to attain the same (or comparable) taste. Usually, that something is sugar or artificial sweeteners, either of which can interfere with metabolism, cause weight gain, and may even be to blame for heart disease. When we eat things that are naturally full of fat, extra sugar and other chemicals aren't needed to make it edible.

Cholesterol Confusion

Fall in love with cholesterol all over again!

Let's talk about that elephant in the room. You may again be wondering what all this healthy fat is going to do to your heart. Take a deep breath. Science has never supported the (false) claims that saturated fat and/or cholesterol cause heart disease. Yet again, the opposite is true.

Heart disease is the leading cause of death in the United States, and still heart health remains one of the most confusing topics in the realm of nutrition. It's also one that's especially personal to me since my own father underwent unexpected major heart surgery not so long ago and because I was first prescribed a statin drug when I was just 20 years young. I remember all too well the feelings of anxiety, helplessness and confusion—having no clue what to do to help my father or myself. At the time, I was studying to become a dietitian (you'd think that would have at least given me an advantage)! After my years of research and experience, I remain confident in my decision to never take that statin drug, and I enjoy a healthy balanced diet which includes eggs cooked in butter practically every morning…which is still shunned by many heart health advocates. I'm confident that I'm not harming my heart, and that I'm actually protecting it with this approach.

You may still be scratching your head at the very thought of including saturated fats like butter and cholesterol-filled egg yolks while you're losing weight. You're not alone in feeling this way. I was confused, too. There are a lot of misconceptions and flat out bad information out there on this topic of heart disease and cholesterol. For years, doctors and dietitians have prescribed a low-fat, low-cholesterol diet (and plenty of statins) for heart health, and coincidentally (or not!), the prevalence of type two diabetes, obesity, cancer and yes, heart disease has skyrocketed!

The good news is that the science is finally being publicized that saturated fat and dietary cholesterol are not linked to heart disease. There was no evidence to support the low-fat message in the first place, nor in generating those guidelines. A group from the American Heart Association and the American College of Cardiology says there is simply not enough evidence to recommend limiting cholesterol in diets (Eckel RH, et al., 2013)[2]. We've been taught to believe that foods manufactured in a laboratory are healthier than real, whole foods from nature, and this is a shame, not to mention flat out dangerous. It's time to make egg white omelettes a thing of the past.

Let's back up for a second. Here's what we've been told: Cholesterol clogs your arteries. It seems to make sense, right? You eat a lot of wax-like cholesterol and flubbery fat and both substances stick to the walls of your arteries and vessels, clogging 'em up and that's what leads to heart disease. Yes?

Not so much.

The reason it's so hard to un-brainwash ourselves of this old, inaccurate way of thinking is because pictures like the one this paints are powerful. It's similar to how easy it is to fall for

---

2   Eckel, RH. "2013 AHA/ACC Guideline on Lifestyle Management to ..." 2013. <https://circ.ahajournals.org/content/early/2013/11/11/01.cir.0000437740.4 8606.d1>

that "fat makes us fat" argument, even though saying "sugar makes us fat" or "carbs make us fat" would be more accurate.

Back to the cholesterol picture—it's wrong because it doesn't work that way. With your internal body temperature being what it is, it wouldn't even be possible for cholesterol to stick to your vessel walls because the flubbery fat and wax-like cholesterol would melt!

The real problem is inflammation. Without inflammation, cholesterol wouldn't accumulate in our vessel walls. It's as if there were a fire and the crew of firefighters came to put out the fire and we blamed them for causing the fire. That would be ridiculous, right? That's exactly what's happening when we blame cholesterol. Cholesterol simply comes to the rescue to heal your body of existing inflammation. So let's not blame the wrong guy. Cholesterol is the hero, not the villain.

A good question is…how did the fire start?

We're learning now that heart disease is truly a sugar disease. Your bread and pasta addiction are likely promoting heart disease—not your eggs or butter. So is your morning bowl of oatmeal with your glass of "heart healthy" orange juice. It can be hard to hear, I know—especially when these foods have been pushed on us for so long as "heart healthy." Think of processed carbs and sugar as little pieces of glass that are cutting up your vessels and causing inflammation. It makes sense as to why pouring fewer shards of glass into your body is beneficial for your heart then, right? Your body needs cholesterol because it uses it to repair those tiny lesions in the blood vessels, which is yet another reason to not fear it!

We now know the key to heart health is to keep internal inflammation at bay by limiting consumption of sugar, grains, processed carbohydrates, and refined oils and eating MORE healthy fats, exercising, managing stress and taking quality, heart protective supplements (which can be found in my free guide that you can download at dietitiancassie.com/ hearthealth). The fact of the matter is that cholesterol and saturated fat do NOT cause heart disease! Replace inflammatory bread and pasta with nutrient-dense veggies and fruits. Replace processed grains that contain anti-nutrients with real food carbohydrates that will protect your heart!

So, let's un-brainwash ourselves and embrace healthy fat, guilt free!

Embrace: Healthy fats are butter, coconut oil, olive oil, avocado oil, cheese, olives, coconut milk (the canned kind), heavy cream, nuts, seeds, nut and seed butters, coconut cream and fat from organic, grass-fed meat. When people recommend lean meat, it's likely because they are assuming you don't have access to high quality meat. If you're getting high quality grass-fed, organic, pasture-raised meat and dairy, I recommend purchasing full fat, both because it's the healthy kind...*and* because it tastes fantastic, too! Since toxins are stored in fat, you'll avoid consuming higher levels of those toxins by choosing lean meat. You can always add good fat in the form of butter, olive oil or avocado.

Speaking of avocado, be friends with the avocado. If you're an "avocado-virgin," that's okay! A lot of my clients are newbies who are afraid of avocados (*How do you know if they're ripe? How do you cut them? How do you eat them?*) Here's the deal: They should feel a bit soft, but not too squishy when you buy them. Avocados have a very short ripeness window, so pick them up at different stages of ripeness from your grocery store. Because they darken as they ripen, get a few dark ones to eat in the next day or two, and then a few green ones to save for later. Keep the green ones on your counter until they turn darker and soften. If you know you won't eat them in the next day or two, put them in the fridge to slow their ripening process. You can cut them with a sharp knife all the way around, open the two halves to expose the pit, and remove it with a stab of your knife or by scooping it out with a spoon. Now you've got two perfect avocado halves! You can serve avocado diced up over a bowl of chili or chicken soup, sliced and over a salad or your scrambled eggs, mashed up in guacamole, or just cut in half and eaten out of the shell with a spoon and some added salt and pepper.

Avoid: I recommend staying away from processed fat sources and man-made oils like canola oil, corn oil, soybean oil, safflower oil, sesame seed oil, cottonseed oil, vegetable oil, shortening and margarine. Also, any oil that has been hydrogenated or partially hydrogenated is a trans fat. If you ever see any oil (even the healthy ones like olive, coconut or avocado) listed as partially hydrogenated or hydrogenated, this is a big, bright, red flag and I recommend staying away from those at all costs. Because of rancidity, oxidation (free radicals), and unhealthy refinement processes, all of these oils can cause inflammation in the body and lead to weight gain. It's also important to keep your oils tightly covered to minimize the damaging effects oxygen has on them. Exposure to oxygen causes oils to become inflammatory. For a similar reason, store oils in a cool, dark place (i.e. no kitchen window sills!).

Portion: A good starting point is including two to three tablespoons of fat every single time you eat—meals, snacks, whenever. This could mean sautéing your veggies in a couple tablespoons of coconut oil at dinner and topping your salad with sliced avocado, or having a heaping spoonful of almond butter on your apple at snack time.

CHAPTER FOUR

THE COLORFUL WORLD
OF CARBS

The C in PFC: Carbs

Okay, we've talked a lot about carbs already, so let's jump in. All carbohydrates, be it pasta, rice, cookies, crackers, even vegetables and fruits, turn into sugar the second they enter your bloodstream. This causes a spike in blood sugar levels, and triggers insulin to be secreted by your pancreas to take care of that sugar—getting it out of your bloodstream and into your cells. That sugar is stored as fat, hence the reason insulin's been dubbed with the infamous title, "fat-storing hormone."

None of this sounds good. Clearly, storing fat won't set you up for success when it comes to your weight loss goal. In fact, it's probably one of the reasons you packed on the pounds in the first place.

So, you may be thinking, "Shouldn't I just skip carbs altogether?" While that would seem to make sense, my answer is a resounding "No!" Here's why: Carbs are the macronutrient that raise your blood sugar levels, which can be a bad thing. However, if you skip them altogether, you'll feel miserable, and that can be just as bad. Protein can be turned into sugar through a process called gluconeogenesis, but that's only if your blood sugar levels get too low due to not eating enough carbohydrates. It's stressful on the body and not something you want it spending its energy and resources on with weight loss as a goal. Just as important as not spiking your blood sugar levels is not letting them drop too low. You want your blood sugars to look like nice rolling hills all day and all night long. The keys to doing that are to not eat too many carbs at once, to balance them out with protein and fat, and to choose the most nutritious forms while avoiding the ones that result in a sugar surge in your bloodstream.

It may take some time and reprogramming of your brain to switch from thinking of carbs as exclusively bread, rice and pasta, and instead, to begin thinking of colorful, nutritious veggies and fruits. I encourage getting most, if not all, of your carbohydrates from veggies and fruits. Think colorful carbs! These real food carbohydrate sources provide more nutrients and antioxidants, and generally they have a far smaller impact on your blood sugar levels, giving you a bigger bang for your buck, so to speak.

No bread? What!? Right. One of the most widely accepted and greatest nutritional misconceptions may be that grains like bread, pasta, rice and cereal are healthy. They've been the base of our food pyramid and the staple foundation of our plate for years. Despite the fact that it's been inGRAINed in our heads that they're healthy, grains can actually bring you further from your weight loss goal than you may realize. I don't recommend grains because of the issues I've seen too many people experience when including them.

When I think of grains, I think of piles of sugar. That's what they are equivalent to. Grains are carbohydrates, so they spike our blood sugar levels, and the problem is that they elicit an insulin response much higher than that of real food carbohydrates like vegetables and even most fruits. With weight loss as your goal, you want to keep the sugar in your bloodstream to a minimum, since it'll end up stored as fat. One slice of bread turns into five or six teaspoons of sugar in your bloodstream, and who has a sandwich with just one slice!? (Remember, you can figure out how many teaspoons of sugar are in any food product by doing the math: A gram of sugar can be hard to picture, but if you divide the number of grams of carbohydrate by four, you get the number of teaspoons of sugar.) Most breads are also packed with junk like corn syrup and trans fats, which send your blood sugar levels skyrocketing and will also cause inflammation in your body.

You've likely been told that if you do not eat bread, you're completely neglecting a food group, and that it's a terrible idea that will only lead to nutrient deficiencies. This is simply not true. Grains contain absolutely nothing—no vitamin, mineral or nutrient—that you can't get from real, whole foods (and just because a food is "whole grain" or "whole wheat" doesn't make it a whole food). Despite what we've been told, grains provide minimal nutritional value and can instead interfere with nutrient absorption due to lectin and phytates, the anti-nutrients they contain. Let's examine these anti-nutrients for a moment.

Nutrient Suckers

Lectins are toxins that are found in all grains and legumes. Like a mushroom that is poisonous, think of lectins as the grain's natural defense that keeps predators away, or makes them sick upon eating too much of it. They wreak havoc on our gut, causing the stomach lining to become inflamed, making it difficult to absorb nutrients in the foods we eat.

Phytates are another toxin found in grains that actually bind to certain nutrients (like iron, zinc, calcium and others) and can slow or inhibit your body's ability to absorb those nutrients. Grains are often "fortified" or "enriched" with vitamins and minerals. This means things like vitamin E, calcium, iron and fiber are added back into the grains after the ingredients have been so highly processed that they are stripped of their nutrients. As amazing as it is that science is able to do that, those vitamins, minerals, and nutrients that are added back in are likely not even absorbed and utilized by your body. Even the "healthiest" kinds, like whole wheat or whole grain bread, are mostly devoid of any kind of real nutrients. Replace bread with vegetables and fruits, and you'll get all of the things grains promise to deliver at a higher concentration *and* without any negative side effects.

"I'll do anything you tell me to, but I'm not giving up my bread." One of my clients, Doug, was eating six slices of bread a day. Two pieces of buttered toast with breakfast, a sandwich at lunch, and two slices spread with peanut butter before bed. "Anything but the bread," he said. I abided by his rule for a little while, but it wasn't sitting right with me. I was doing him a disservice by not being more firm with my no-bread recommendation, especially because he wasn't reaching his weight loss goal as quickly as he wanted to.

"I just don't see the big deal. I don't drink pop, I don't eat candy, and I don't even eat chips, crackers, or cookies. It's hard to believe that saying goodbye to bread would magically make the pounds disappear." As hard as it may have been to believe, that was indeed the case, and once Doug reluctantly humored me, he got to experience it firsthand.

Grains & Gluten

Lots of grains—including wheat, rye and barley—contain the protein gluten. While I stressed the importance of *quality* protein earlier, it's important to note that there is no such thing as *quality* gluten. This is because, unfortunately, most digestive systems do not digest gluten well. As a result, it can be responsible for weight gain due to potential food sensitivities and their interference with nutrient absorption, and it causes an inflammatory response in your body. In fact, many people are sensitive to gluten even if their symptoms are not as aggressive or inflammatory as you may see in someone with Celiac Disease—an autoimmune condition and the most serious form of gluten intolerance. When somebody with celiac disease consumes gluten, their cells try to attack the gluten, and in the process, they attack the rest of the body at the same time, causing serious internal damage. The only known solution for celiac disease is to simply avoid anything with gluten.

The tricky reality is that you can be sensitive to gluten without having full blown celiac disease, and a lot of people are. This is a real problem with real symptoms and real consequences if you continue to consume gluten when you are sensitive to it. When you are sensitive to gluten and ingest it, an inflammatory reaction takes place in your body. The reaction significantly varies from person to person, and it can manifest itself in a wide variety of symptoms. Many of our clients find that gluten is the cause of their bloating, diarrhea, constipation, cramping, headaches, skin conditions, acid reflux, joint and muscle pain, rashes, ulcers, depression, allergies and so many other things. After removing it for a period of time, their symptoms disappear and when they introduce it again, these symptoms come back.

Some people who are gluten sensitive are asymptomatic, meaning they don't exhibit symptoms, at least for a certain period of their lives. This is why it's possible for symptoms to suddenly appear out of nowhere. It's no wonder so many of our clients say things like "But I've been eating bread my whole life without any problems…so it can't be the bread." It could be! Sometimes the negative consequences from a lifetime of eating lots of bread (anyone else do this while on a low-fat diet?) can catch up later in life, either through a slowed metabolism or weight that simply won't drop.

There's plenty of research to support that non-celiac gluten sensitivity does exist, so I don't feel the need to repeat that all here. The fact of the matter is that no one needs gluten, and we're all better off without it. So you've got nothing to lose when it comes to ditching the grains. To me, it's not worth it to consume a processed carbohydrate when there are so many delicious, nutritious, real food carbohydrates that will support you in feeling and looking your best. When in doubt, keep it simple and opt for real, unprocessed food. Pay attention to your body and how it responds to certain foods. My PFC-balanced approach is naturally gluten free! It doesn't need to be complicated.

So do you have to give up bread? The choice is yours. I'm not making you do anything! When it comes down to it, I vow to always keep it simple. I don't recommend bread, dinner rolls, grains, or pasta. You don't need them. If you listen closely to your body, it will always tell you to choose the vegetables and fruits over the English muffin or bagel. I suggest replacing bread with lettuce wraps and pasta with spaghetti squash. Keep the focus on vegetables and fruits for carbs, and you'll find that you aren't missing out on anything. It doesn't hurt to try foregoing the grains for a few days to see how you feel. You may be pleasantly surprised!

This was the case for Doug. When he ditched it, those stubborn pounds began to disappear, and so did his cravings for bread. After just a week, he completely lost interest in bread, which had previously accompanied his every meal. He was astonished, and it was well worth it to him to breakup with the bread forever to achieve the health and weight loss he had so long sought after.

The Grain Drain

Julie was falling asleep at her desk every afternoon by 3pm. "I figured it was because I was overworked and not sleeping enough. But it turned out that my biggest problem was the bread. Who knew!?" Once Julie ditched bread and grains, she not only had the energy to make it through her work day, but she was also able to add in a workout on top of it! The bread at lunch had been making her sleepy and adding to her waistline. Parting with the bread resulted in shedding the pounds while experiencing sustained energy.

"But I love peanut butter sandwiches!" you may say. Do you know what else loves peanut butter? Apples. Celery loves it too. Think outside of the box. Try giving up bread for one week and see how you feel. Once you realize you can make it a week, try for another. Replace your bread and grains with vegetables and fruits—enjoy lettuce wraps with tuna or chicken salad, a sweet potato with your dinner instead of the dinner roll, and add a bunch of spinach to your eggs in the morning and skip the toast! When you realize how much better you feel, you won't be tempted to stroll down the bread aisle again. You may find that while initially it seems like an impossible task, you feel so great after eliminating it that you may never want to eat grains again. If you do eat them again, it's a good idea to pay attention to how you feel when you reintroduce them into your body. Don't be surprised if you experience sluggishness, cravings, headaches or even weight gain, like Doug, Julie and so many of our other clients have as a result of bread and grains.

As always, keeping it simple with real food and the PFC method is the way to go! However, if you do choose to include grains, I'd suggest going for gluten-free ones, like rice and gluten-free oatmeal, and make sure they are PFC-balanced (mix protein powder and butter in with your oatmeal and serve your rice with chicken and avocado or cashews). This is a better alternative to the gluten grains, but the downfall is that gluten-free grains still cause inflammation because they still turn to sugar. So remember, if you find yourself still stuck with those stubborn pounds after following the rest of the recommendations in this book, you may want to revisit ditching your grains.

Also, as you eat more fat and protein with your carbs, you'll notice your desire for carbs and sugar decreasing. This is because when you eat carbs, you don't receive a message to stop eating until your stomach is physically stretched and full. When you eat fats and proteins, they help slow the digestion of carbs in addition to sending your brain a hormonal message (cholecystokinin) telling you to stop eating. That's why when you eat a banana by itself, it doesn't fill you up, and an hour later, you may even be hungrier than you were before you ate it. When you eat half of that banana, with a handful of nuts for fat and a hard-boiled egg or beef stick for protein, you balance your blood sugars and in turn, feel more stable overall. The protein and fat help to keep you more satisfied until your next meal or snack, whereas if you had a carbohydrate by itself you might be ravished in an hour or two.

Your Carb Sweet Spot

When it comes to protein and fat, the portion sizes I recommend for you as a starting point are based on what I've found works for the majority of of my clients—and those amounts don't vary much. Now, carbs are a totally different story. Because carbohydrates have the greatest effect on your blood sugar levels, it's necessary to find your personal sweet spot in order to get your weight in check. Once you find your carb sweet spot, you'll basically be filling in the gaps with healthy fat (at least two tablespoons, but you may find you feel better and lose weight quicker with more). Let me explain.

Many of my clients see the results they're after for their waistlines and energy levels when following my general recommended portion sizes for carbs (a couple cups of non-starchy carbs and a half a cup of starchy carbs or fruit—I explain the difference between starchy carbs and non-starchy carbs at the very end of this chapter) at every meal and snack. That said, sometimes these amounts need to be adjusted and monitored in order to nail that sweet spot so that you can really start shedding the pounds.

When it comes to finding your optimal carbohydrate intake, the best way to go about it is trial and error. Your carb sweet spot is the place where your energy levels are sustained, your sugar cravings are gone, and the weight is coming off.

When I talk about the carbohydrate sweet spot, two clients come to mind: Jane and Jackie. Both of these women came to me around the same time and they both had some high weight loss goals. My initial recommendation for both of them was a cup or two of non-starchy carbs, along with a half cup of either starchy veggies or fruit at every meal and snack. Over time, we continuously adjusted that amount based on their hunger levels, cravings, energy levels, and weight loss. The results were very interesting.

First off, with Jane, we ended up finding out that she was more sensitive to carbohydrates. The pounds didn't start dropping until we reduced her portions of starchy carbs to a quarter cup and completely cut out fruit. This helped reduce her sugar cravings, making it easier for her to stay on track with her PFC-balanced eating and weight loss. Half a cup of starchy carbs and even a piece of fruit were too much for Jane's body to handle—that small amount was sending her for a ride on the blood sugar roller coaster. It made sense why she wasn't feeling great or losing weight until we reduced the starchy carbs.

On the other hand, with Jackie, we found that she needed to up her carb intake to nearly a cup of starchy veggies or a whole piece of fruit at meals and snacks in order to get her metabolism revved up to the point where it was burning fat and she was losing weight. We discovered this to be the case because she had come in with low energy levels, headaches, and sugar cravings. They didn't improve until we increased her carb intake. Once we did that, she felt like a new woman!

Now, Jane and Jackie are different women with different biochemistries, genetics, lifestyles and health histories. Of course, it makes sense that what worked for Jane wouldn't necessarily be the same for Jackie. That's why what works for your friend, spouse, co-worker or someone else reading this book, may not necessarily be what works for you. The best way to find out is to pick a starting point and experiment by increasing your carbs for a couple days, and then reducing them for a couple days, until you find your own sweet spot, just as Jane and Jackie did. When you do find your carbohydrate sweet spot, stick with it along with my recommend portions of protein, and fill in the rest with healthy fat.

Embrace: Vegetables and some fruit. Vegetables can be divided into two categories: starchy and non-starchy. Starchy vegetables like corn, peas, beets, squash, yams, sweet potatoes and plantains are denser and have a greater effect on blood sugar levels. Non-starchy vegetables like broccoli, cauliflower, cabbage, kale, peppers, green beans, cucumbers, and asparagus hardly raise your blood sugar levels, if at all. Fruit is generally on the same playing field as starchy vegetables, depending on the type of fruit. Berries and citrus fruits have less of an impact on blood sugar levels than bananas, apples, and pears.

For weight loss, the non-starchy vegetables are the carbohydrate group I recommend eating most over the others because they impact your blood sugar levels the least. When watching your waistline, you'll want to watch your fruit and starchy carb intake. Although full of nutrients, antioxidants, fiber and phytonutrients, fruit and starchy carbs turn into a lot more sugar than the non-starchy carbs. If you're choosing fruit or a starch as your carbohydrate choice at most meals and snacks, then this could make it harder for your body to lose weight. Keep it simple and opt for non-starchy veggies like broccoli, asparagus, peppers, spinach, kale and cauliflower most of the time.

Avoid: Grains, pasta, bread, rice, cereal, muffins, cakes, cookies, pretzels, chips and any and all other processed, refined carbohydrates which take your blood sugar levels for a roller coaster ride, contribute to inflammation, and take you further from your metabolism and weight loss goals. Reducing your consumption of sugar and processed foods is a great way to avoid the blood sugar roller coaster altogether. These are foods that have been chemically processed and made from refined ingredients.

Think about it like this: if you don't have the ingredients in your kitchen, and if you couldn't fathom how it is possibly created, then it's probably a processed food. Processed foods are generally high in carbohydrates AND trans fats, which we talked about staying away from in the last chapter. Processed foods will never be able to compete with the nutrients we receive from whole foods. Strive to eat like your great grandparents by staying away from packaged and processed foods, and do your best to get your carbohydrates from vegetables and fruits.

Portion: In general, sticking to a half cup of starchy vegetables or fruit is a good place to start. With non-starchy vegetables like broccoli, cauliflower, spinach and cucumbers, the portion size is pretty much unlimited since they hardly have any impact on your blood sugar levels. In fact, because they are somewhat difficult to break down, they may even require more energy to process than we even receive from them. This means we gain important nutrients without a blood sugar spike, and for that reason I suggest that you fill up on these first (shoot for a couple cups at each meal!). Limit the starchier veggies and fruit to about a half cup (or even a quarter cup) at a time to help prevent blood sugar spikes. A quarter cup may seem rigid if you're used to snacking on fruit, but if losing weight is your goal, it's important to minimize the sugar you're consuming and choose non-starchy veggies for your carbs as much as possible. If you pick carbohydrates from the ones I recommend avoiding, try to stick with a half cup, or a single slice of bread to limit their impact.

CHAPTER FIVE

WHERE DOES DAIRY FIT?

Now, I know this book is about forgetting restriction and eating what your body needs (no more calorie counting and eat healthy fat for heaven's sake!). At the same time, it's about unlocking stubborn weight loss, and I'd be doing you a disservice if I didn't tell you about a food category that could be standing right between you and your weight loss goal: Dairy.

You may already be wondering how dairy fits into PFC-balanced eating. If you choose to include dairy in your diet, it can count as your fat and carbohydrate source, so long as you're getting full fat dairy (which is what I recommend). That said, dairy is a gray area, and I don't recommend all dairy products. My two main concerns with dairy are that a lot of people are sensitive to it and it is also a strong promoter of weight gain. I'll elaborate on this further when we discuss food sensitivities in Chapter Eight.

The reason dairy promotes weight gain is because it is particularly "insulinogenic." That's a big word. When you break it down, it essentially means stimulating the production of insulin. I'm sure at this point you're familiar with insulin, your fat-storing hormone. So basically this means that dairy elicits a surprisingly high insulin response, causing you to secrete lots and lots of insulin, and in turn your body stores lots and lots of fat. End result: When you consume dairy, you pack on the pounds.

Now, don't get mad at dairy. It does what it is actually supposed to do. Dairy products, whether they're from cows, sheep or goats, contain hormones and factors that help baby mammals grow. Just like breast milk promotes a baby human's growth, cow's milk helps baby cows grow, sheep's milk helps baby sheep grow and goat's milk helps baby goats grow. It makes sense for babies that need to grow, but not so much for an adult like yourself looking to lose weight.

The good news here is that certain dairy products, such as heavy cream, butter and hard cheeses are *not* very insulinogenic, so while these are considered dairy products, they get a free pass in this discussion. (Milk, yogurt and cottage cheese do fall into this insulinogenic category of dairy products.) That's not to say you couldn't be sensitive to heavy cream, butter or cheese, but it's less likely than the others I mentioned. We'll discuss this further a few more chapters in.

Whether you are sensitive to dairy or not, consuming dairy products will cause your body to produce more insulin, which causes you to store more body fat. We see clients with stalled weight loss goals who jump-start their weight loss by cutting out most, if not all, dairy products.

Now, you might be wondering how you will get your calcium without dairy in your diet. Calcium is a commonly misunderstood nutrient. The truth of the matter is since dairy is so difficult to digest, most of us don't actually absorb much of the calcium contained in it (especially if we have poor gut health, as I will outline in Chapter Seven). Besides, calcium isn't just in dairy products. A healthy intestinal tract will allow you to absorb calcium found in plenty of other non-dairy foods, such as seafood (like salmon and scallops), leafy greens (like spinach, kale and broccoli), nuts, sesame seeds...even tap water contains calcium. For comparison purposes, a cup of skim milk contains 300mg of calcium, and so does four and a half ounces of canned salmon or a cup and a half of collard greens. Most of us are actually getting plenty of calcium and for that reason, you won't find it anywhere in my guide with the most important supplements (which you can download at dietitiancassie.com/supplements).

You don't need dairy. Your waistline will be better without it. If you do choose to include it, ideally you're choosing raw, organic, unpasteurized grass-fed sources. Most conventionally raised cows are kept confined in a small area, fed a diet that they are not accustomed to eating (cows eat grass, not corn and grain. We've also heard of claims of leftover holiday candy, orange peels, and whatever they can scrape up from the bottom of a chicken coop...yuck!) Because of this junk, they eventually find themselves with weakened immune systems. Just like in humans, a weakened immune system can lead to cow sickness. To prevent this, many farmers add antibiotics to their chow, along with hormones necessary for increased and extended milk production. This means that if you're purchasing conventional dairy products, you're getting higher than normal levels of these contaminants. Not good. That's why if you do choose to include dairy, it's a smart idea to pick up the highest quality milk you can find. Raw, grass-fed, organic, unpasteurized dairy is the gold standard. Do your best to find something close to this. There are many local farmers who will sell you high quality dairy if you head out to their farms, or join their farm's dairy cooperative. Otherwise, make the best selection from what your co-op or grocery store offers. Note: Local laws may prevent sales of raw dairy products—in that case, find something grass fed and/or organic.

Remember how Doug in the last chapter didn't want to give up his bread but once he did, he began dropping pounds left and right? In Chapter Eight, I'll share a similar story about Emily who experienced similar results when she ditched the dairy. You get to decide what you're willing to do, or not. Ultimately, it all boils down to your goals. If your goal is weight loss, then I encourage you to take a break from the dairy products and see what happens. Again, many people do not realize dairy is a problem for them until they cut it out for a few weeks, so if you haven't done a dairy-free experiment, I encourage you to do so. What do you have to lose (other than those stubborn pounds)? You can download my free guide on how to go dairy-free at dietitiancassie.com/dairy.

CHAPTER SIX

HERE'S YOUR GAME PLAN

Now that you know your PFC's, let's put 'em all together, starting with your very first meal of the day.

Jumpstart Your Metabolism

I recommend starting the day on a strong note by eating within an hour of the alarm clock sounding to "jumpstart" your metabolism. Breakfast is the most important meal of the day! That's a common phrase we've all heard, and for good reason. The word *breakfast* breaks down into two words: "break" and "fast," because breakfast is the meal that breaks your overnight fast. After sleeping for hours, eating breakfast is a tried and true way to "jumpstart" your metabolism first thing in the morning because breakfast brings your blood sugar levels back into the stable range. Don't miss this opportunity to kick your metabolism into gear!

The problem with typical breakfast foods like cereal with skim milk, oatmeal, toast, pancakes, waffles, bagels, fruit and orange juice is that it's a carb BOMB waiting to go off a couple hours later. Then that mid-morning pick-me-up snack of a mocha and muffin or maybe a banana if you're trying to be healthy is another carb bomb that spikes your blood sugars, which then rapidly drop, and you wonder why you're hungrier an hour later than before you even had that snack. We've been told that these highly processed, high-carbohydrate foods are healthy, but they contain little, if any, protein and fat to counterbalance the sugar they are digested as the second they enter your body, and that's why you crash and burn shortly after.

You need fat and protein to balance your blood sugar and keep you stable throughout the day. The best breakfast of all is a couple eggs (protein) cooked in butter or coconut oil (fat) with a side of sautéed sweet potato or fruit (carbs). Dinner leftovers work great if you're not a "breakfast eater" (breakfast food doesn't need to be "breakfast food!" Who came up with special foods for the morning, anyway?) So, you can keep the pilot light of your metabolism furnace going first thing in the morning with a PFC-balanced breakfast, or you can blow out the pilot (dangerous!) before your day even starts by having dessert for breakfast. I recommend the former!

If you're not hungry or if you're in a hurry, it's still important to eat, and in both of these cases I recommend making a protein smoothie. This is a simple, quick way to get in your P, F and C. Blend a couple scoops of protein powder with a healthy fat like half an avocado, a couple tablespoons of nut butter or a quarter cup of coconut milk and the carbs of your choice, such as a handful of frozen berries or half a banana. Blend with ice and water to your desired consistency. My favorite PFC-balanced smoothie recipe can be found at dietitiancassie.com/smoothie.

PFC Every Three

After breakfast, try to space out your eating to every three to four hours for the rest of the day, ending on a strong note with a bedtime snack about a half hour before bed. (A WHAT?! Trust me on this. In fact, the bedtime snack is SO key that it has it's very own chapter where I'll elaborate on exactly why you need to incorporate it into your routine in order for your weight loss to happen).

It doesn't matter if you wake up early or sleep in late—simply eat within an hour of waking and then every few hours after that. The reasoning for this is that it is a way to stay ahead of your hunger so that your blood sugar levels remain stable throughout the day. This keeps glucagon (your fat-burning hormone) working in your favor so you can shed the pounds. If you're a former dieter, you may find this has you eating more often than you're used to. Keep in mind that your meals and snacks don't have to be large—your goal is to keep your hunger around a 5 (on a scale of 1 to 10). If you're not super hungry, you can eat less at that meal or snack, but I'd strongly urge you not to skip it. (Skipping it is a surefire way to let your blood sugar levels drop too low.) Many of our clients have found it helpful to set an alarm on their phone to remind them when it's time to eat, since it can be easy to get caught up in a project or activity and not remember to eat until you feel like you're "starving." At that point, your metabolism has already slowed down! Make it a priority to eat "PFC Every Three" to keep your metabolism high and to stay in fat-burning mode and it'll become a habit in no time!

Rules of the Game

▶ Try not to count

Holding on to old ways of thinking while trying to follow my PFC-balanced eating regimen is a recipe for disaster. No calculators around here! If you're counting, you're probably restricting, which means you're not fueling your body with what it needs to run most efficiently and be a fat-burning machine. Everything changes when you see food in a brand new light, as something that nourishes and fuels your body, instead of something to deprive yourself from. It's crucial to completely let go of your former dieting mindset and un-brainwash yourself from obsessing over the amounts of food or calories you are taking in. Focus on establishing a healthy relationship with your body, nourishing it by eating lots of quality protein, healthy fats, and nutrient-dense carbohydrates. Your metabolism will heal, you will get back in touch with your "hunger sensor," and your body will regulate itself as it should, and in turn, the pounds will melt away.

▶ Don't blow it on beverages

The saddest way to negate your healthy eating efforts is with sugar-laden beverages. Drinking water is your best bet. Try carbonated water, coconut water, and drink plenty of filtered water during the day to stay hydrated. This helps your body with its natural detoxification process so that it can excrete chemicals and toxins that drag your metabolism down. To determine the minimum amount of water you should consume each day, take half of your body weight in pounds and simply change it to ounces (i.e. a 150 pound person should drink 75 ounces of water). It's also a good idea to invest in a water filter because many chemicals, like chlorine and fluoride, are in our water systems. As an alternative, club soda (or seltzer water or soda water—it's all the same) is a refreshing sugar and artificial sweetener-free option; it's my go-to at restaurants. Unsweetened tea and coffee (black or with heavy cream, butter, almond milk or coconut milk) are good options too! Now, when it comes to wine, remember, it can add up fast. I like wine as much as the next person, but if you don't believe me, just read Chapter Eighteen to see how it blocked Lisa's weight loss goal.

Now, just to be clear, these other suggestions aren't to be had in place of water (common sense should say drinking half your body weight in coffee is a terrible idea!), but rather as supplementary options on how to mix things up a bit.

▶ **Pay attention to portions**

How much of each group should you eat? While I don't recommend counting points, calories, grams or anything else, it is important to be aware of portion sizes. Because this isn't a one-size-fits-all approach, how much you need may differ from my general recommendations found in this book. Let your body tell you what it needs. Past dieting has taught us to completely disregard our hunger signals. Let's work on getting back in touch with these important cues. At meal time, a good starting point is four to six ounces of protein (equivalent to about the thickness and circumference of the palm of your hand), a couple tablespoons of fat, a half cup of starchy carbs and/or several cups of non-starchy ones. At snacks, you're looking at about half of those amounts.

Your goal is to not feel starved or stuffed—follow Goldilocks' advice: aim for, "Juuuuust right." On a hunger scale of 1 to 10, you should stay between a 4 and a 6 at all times. If you can't make it to your next meal or snack because you're hungry, then by all means, eat! The goal is to fuel your body and don't forget that when you're hungry, your metabolism is already slowing down to compensate. Your metabolism doesn't function if you don't feed it. Aim to keep it turbocharged at all times for weight loss and peak energy. So, when hungry, eat a PFC-balanced snack and make a mental note that next time you need to eat more. If you're still full after four hours have passed, then next time you should eat less. Make connections by noticing how different foods affect your mood, energy levels and cravings, and pay attention to how you feel if you happen to leave out a macronutrient (a P, F or C).

If you are eating consistently throughout the day with PFC-balanced meals and snacks, your body will tell you when to stop. Pay attention to it, and honor it. Real foods help normalize your body's satiety mechanisms and prevent cravings and binge eating by keeping blood sugar levels stable throughout the day. Pay attention to your portions, but don't overanalyze it.

Here are a few things to consider when thinking about your portion sizes:

- Do you have a form of protein, fat, and carbs on your plate?

- Is your protein about the size of the palm of your hand?

- Do you have at least two tablespoons of fats on your plate?

- Are you keeping your intake of starchy vegetables or fruit at a half cup serving and/or having a cup or two of non-starchy veggies?

- Are you subconsciously still cutting calories or fat? Make sure you are eating enough! Many people still have that low-fat mindset when buttering their broccoli and hold back on the fats, or even worse, skip meals. Un-brainwash yourself!

- Has it been more than a few hours since you've eaten? If so, try having a small snack while you're preparing dinner so you don't gorge yourself at mealtime.

Just to recap: Many of the foods we eat fall into more than one of the PFC categories. In general, I consider something to be P, F or C based on whichever macronutrient the food contains the most of. You can look at the nutrition facts label on packaged food to find this information. Keep in mind the protein choices that support metabolism most are animal products, like meat, fish, and eggs. Therefore, I count foods like peanut butter or cheese, (both of which contain fat AND protein) as fats—not only do they have more fat than protein, but they aren't proteins that support metabolism the most. When in doubt, count the food as whichever macro it has most of and don't stress about it too much! Again, it's not about perfection, it's about eating as balanced as you can.

▶ **Consistency Beats Perfection**

Most importantly, know that it's *not* about perfection. As much as I dislike counting calories, I dislike getting nitty-gritty about eating even more. Too often, I see clients put off making healthy changes because they know they won't be militant. They have one bad snack and let it turn into a bad day. Or one bad day and let it turn into a bad week or even month. This is devastating, and it certainly doesn't need to be this way! Don't let your fear of not being perfect interfere with being a healthier you.

While it's important to set out to do the best that you can, setting your expectations too high can lead to a sense of failure and frustration. Do the best that you can as often as you can and don't worry about the rest. There's no need to be super rigid—it's all about listening to your body, eating when you're hungry, stopping when you're full and paying attention to how you feel when you skip a P, F or C, or eat one of the foods I recommend avoiding. Keep the focus on eating real food in balance and learn to listen to your body. Even when you aren't perfect, when you strive to eat in PFC balance, you'll still feel great.

Of far greater importance than perfection is consistency...even on the weekends. In order for your body to trust you enough to burn what you put into it, you need to be consistent. I've seen enough clients try the weekday consistency thing, and have a free-for-all on the weekend. Often times, this means kicking off the weekend with a Thursday evening Happy Hour. (We'll touch on Happy Hours in Chapter Eighteen.) When you do the math, if you're off your game Thursday night through Sunday, then that's forty-three percent of the time! I wouldn't trust someone who's inconsistent nearly half of the time, and your body isn't any different when it comes to trusting you. It won't trust you to fuel it with the right foods at the right times unless you're proving that you can do just that most of the time. Skipping days is how habits fall apart. Of course you won't be perfect, and again, that's not the expectation. But, if you're serious about your weight loss goal, then it's essential to do the best that you can with your "PFC Every Three" most of the time. You are training your body to be a fat-burning machine, so giving it the same message over and over again is what's going to get it, and your weight, to where you want it to be.

Don't forget that the choice is yours and the suggestions here are simply *recommendations.* They are meant to keep you off the blood sugar roller coaster so that you can lose weight! Of course, balance is individualized and finding your balance is something only you can do. Find the way of eating that makes you feel your best and your most balanced self by considering what I've found to work and giving it a whirl. Do your best to include a P, F and C every time you eat! The closer you can eat all three components of PFC together, the better. At minimum, try to always have a source of protein or healthy fat with your carbohydrate to promote balanced blood sugar levels. A good rule of thumb is to never eat a carbohydrate alone, but since it's not about perfection, do your best and try to at least have some protein and fat when you do have a carb. You'll get the hang of it soon enough.

Examples of PFC-Balanced Meals and Snacks:

A meal might look like:

- 2-3 scrambled eggs (P) cooked in 2 tablespoons of butter (F) + 2 cups spinach + 1/2 cup sautéed sweet potato (C)

- 1 cup of salmon salad made with 3-4 ounces wild Alaskan salmon (P) + 2-3 tablespoons full fat mayonnaise (F) + 1/2 cup chopped celery and 1/2 cup grapes (PFC)

- 4 ounces of steak strips (P) stir fried in 2 tablespoons of coconut oil (F) + 1-2 cups mixed vegetables (broccoli, cauliflower, celery, green beans, carrots, water chestnuts) served over 1/2 cup spaghetti squash noodles (C)

- 5 ounces of grilled chicken (P) + 1/2 avocado sliced + 1 ounce feta cheese + 1 Tablespoon sunflower seeds (F) over 3 cups of leafy greens + 1/2 diced apple + 1/2 cup halved tomatoes +1/2 cup sliced cucumbers (C)

- 4 ounce grass-fed beef burger (P) + 1 tablespoon pumpkin seeds + 5-10 olives (F) served over 1 cup fresh greens topped with 1/2 cup mixed vegetables (tomato, cucumber) (FC) + a side of 1/2 cup cooked carrots (C)

- 6 ounces of wild Alaskan salmon (P) drizzled with 2 tablespoons of butter (F) on top of 2 cups of spinach + 1/2 sweet potato (C)

- Balanced smoothie with 1 scoop whey protein powder (P) + ¼ cup coconut milk (F) + 1 cup spinach + 1/2 cup blueberries (C)

A snack might look like:

- ½ cup tuna salad made with 2 ounces white albacore tuna (P) + 2 tablespoons olive oil (F) + ½ cup raspberries (C)

- 1-2 hard boiled eggs (P) + 2 tablespoons nut butter (F) + ½ banana (C)

- 1-2 ounces grilled chicken (P) + 2 tablespoons full fat cream cheese (F) + a pickle (C)

- 1 ounce dried beef stick (P) + guacamole (1/2 avocado with fresh squeezed lime and diced tomatoes) (F) + 2-3 cups raw veggies (C)

- 1 deviled egg made with 1 hardboiled egg (P) + 2 tablespoons full fat mayonnaise (F) + a clementine (C)

- 1 slice of egg bake consisting of 1-2 eggs (P) + 1-2 tablespoons butter (F) + chopped veggies (C)

You can download my free Getting Started Guide which includes these lists of the PFC categories for your reference at dietitiancassie.com/PFC.

PART 2

THE UNSEEN OBSTACLES
IN THE WAY OF
YOUR WEIGHT LOSS

CHAPTER SEVEN

TIME FOR A GUT CHECK

When it comes to evaluating your stubborn weight loss, a critical and often overlooked factor is the gut—the place where digestion, absorption, and elimination all happen. Oddly, most practitioners completely overlook the gut. With our clients, we've found it to be a key starting point for general health and weight loss. Gut health goes well beyond gas, bloating, or emergency bathroom trips. Practically everything about your body is tied to the gut, including your weight. The old saying holds true: "Health begins in the gut."

You can eat the "right foods," but if you aren't digesting them properly, you aren't going to see the progress you want because your body still won't be getting the nutrients it needs. *Eating* healthy food is only half of the nutrition equation— you also need to be in the ideal state to *digest* it. So, while it's important to make the best food choices possible, it's just as important to help your body digest them. After working with thousands of clients, I've found that most of us have varying levels of impaired gut health. The good news is that you can improve it! Before we get into that, let's explore what "gut health" even means.

What's Gut Health?

The term gut health covers digestion and absorption of food and immune status; it's the cornerstone of achieving optimal health, and the avenue through which nutrients are absorbed, assimilated, and incorporated into the body. Gut health is associated with every other process, system, organ, and cell in your body! In the same way that our solar system revolves around the sun, your bodily systems revolve around your gut. Your gut is where your metabolism starts, food is digested, and nutrients are absorbed.

Scientists recently began calling your gut your "second brain." This is because your neurotransmitters (brain chemicals) are made in your gut, which means your gut and brain are intricately connected. Long before the research supported this connection, this link has been apparent as we may get a stomach ache when we are anxious—a possible origin of the phrase, "I have a gut feeling." This adds new, truer meaning to the phrase, "You are what you eat" more than ever before.

On top of everything else, your gut serves as the fighting grounds where good bacteria keep foreign invaders at bay. Your gut is a barrier to toxins and pathogens, and about 70% of your immune system is located there.

Now, normally you may not pay much attention to your gut health—you're not alone. Because your digestive system may be the single most important factor in reclaiming your health, it actually could be the key to unlocking that stubborn weight loss! Whether or not your gut is healthy will determine how your digestion functions, how likely you are to have cravings, how energetic you feel, how well your immune system works, and whether you're gaining or losing pounds. If your gut health isn't up to par, even the most nutritious foods may not be broken down or absorbed properly. So while it is important to make the best food choices possible, it is just as important to be in the proper state to digest that food. Your gut health goal is to create an environment where gut bacteria are living in harmony and taking care of you as they should. Now let's talk about how your gut can become unhealthy.

Inflammation's Role in Gut Health

Poor gut health can be a result of a multitude of lifestyle factors, including:

- Sugar and processed foods (like candy, cookies, hot dogs and french fries)
- Refined carbohydrates (like bread, pasta, cereal, crackers, cookies, granola bars, muffins, bagels, pretzels and chips)
- Processed vegetable oils (canola, soybean, corn, sunflower and rapeseed)
- Artificial sweeteners
- Alcohol
- Antibiotic use
- Eating poorly raised conventional meat
- Taking poor quality supplements
- Chronic Stress
- Overexercise
- Food sensitivities (like gluten or dairy)

All of these factors are problematic because they can lead to bodywide inflammation. New research is pointing to inflammation as the root cause of almost *all* weight gain. In addition to that, inflammation can cause heart disease, type-2 diabetes, and even cancer.

At this point, you might be wondering whether you're supposed to be focusing on inflammation or gut health. Well, healing the gut and tackling inflammation go hand in hand—you can't have a healthy gut if you don't first address inflammation.

How do you know you have inflammation? Clues that you may have chronic inflammation are chronic fatigue, being overweight and difficulty losing weight, sugar cravings, chronic aches and pains, constipation, diarrhea, indigestion, dry skin, acne, psoriasis, and allergies. In order to know if these symptoms are being caused by inflammation, you should know the various types of inflammation.

There are two main types of inflammation: one that's good and one that's bad. Let's dive into distinguishing the differences between them, and take an in-depth look at how we can avoid or heal the bad inflammation that we don't want.

The first type, acute inflammation, is probably what comes to mind when you hear the word "inflammation." You stub your toe, you get a cut or a burn, or maybe a black eye. Your body's natural inflammatory response is redness, warmth, swelling, and maybe even loss of function or pain.

This acute inflammation is normal and necessary—it's your body's innate mechanism to help protect and heal itself—so it's a good thing. Think of it like a fire truck at the scene of a fire. They put out the fire and continue on to the next fire. But, what happens if that first fire keeps getting bigger? What happens when *all* the fire trucks are focusing on that one fire? Well, if a fire breaks out somewhere else, there aren't going to be any available fire trucks left because they're all held up at the first scene. That means the second fire will continue to do more damage and get more out of control until the first fire is put out.

Now, don't get me wrong: acute inflammation isn't a problem. The inflammatory response starts up when needed, and then dies down once it has done its job—that's normal. The fire truck arrived at the scene, extinguished the fire, and returned to the fire station to await the next call. It's when your body loses its ability to turn off the inflammatory response and it stops being an acute response and remains a constantly engaged, low grade, systemic response...that's when it becomes an issue. Enter chronic inflammation.

When chronic inflammation occurs, it starts damaging healthy tissue in your body. What started out as a small fire grew out of control, gradually burning down the entire forest. Chronic inflammation is a scary thing, especially because the symptoms aren't obvious. It manifests itself in different ways from one person to another. In one person, inflammation may show up as heart disease, in another person as acne, and in another as obesity. Chronic inflammation contributes to everything from achy joints to asthma to irritable bowel disease to diabetes to heart disease to migraines to skin rashes—the list goes on. Your body sees it as a fire and is always going to prioritize taking care of the inflammation before anything else. This means that if you want to lose weight, it's going to be really tough for your body to achieve that without first reducing inflammation.

What most people don't know is that inflammation stems from the gut. That's why the gut becomes such a critical starting point, and healing the inflammation is key to getting on track to weight loss. So how do you do that?

Here is my three-step approach to tackling inflammation, thus healing your gut and getting you on your way to hitting your weight loss goals.

Step 1: Stop Causing Damage

The first step we take with all of our clients is to have them stop causing additional damage to their already inflamed gut by removing inflammatory triggers. This is basically everything from the list I outlined earlier which outlines foods that directly cause and/or promote inflammation. Let's dig into each one. Just a heads up, most of these get their own upcoming chapter because they're just that important. I'll take the time now to foreshadow.

Sugar Intake

Keeping sugar intake low and focusing on avoiding refined carbohydrates, added sugar, and processed foods is imperative because these damage the lining in your gut and create an environment in which bad bacteria can thrive. By consuming these, you are essentially feeding the bad bacteria and allowing them to multiply. In addition, grains and processed, refined foods can be hard to digest and cause perforations in your intestines. Think of sugar as little pieces of glass that cut up your vessels and cause inflammation. That includes cookies, crackers, bread, pasta, oats, and even brown rice. It's important to work hard at reducing consumption of these foods—at least for the duration of the healing process, and hopefully in the long-term as well.

Artificial Sweeteners

All artificial sweeteners (also known as sugar substitutes)—saccharin, sucralose (commonly known as Splenda), aspartame—they're all artificial and they all have some serious consequences associated with their consumption, including negatively impacting our gut health by killing off the good bacteria. When that happens, your gut can be damaged and inflammation occurs—the last thing you want if you're trying to lose weight. We will look at a whole chapter on artificial sweeteners later. For now, instead of these, I suggest using pure stevia, which is a natural sweetener that comes from a plant, not a lab.

Alcohol

Alcohol consumption can wreak havoc on your gut, and for this, along with other reasons we'll cover later on in Chapter Eighteen, keeping alcohol intake to a minimum—if not removing it completely—is essential for your weight loss goal.

Antibiotics

Antibiotics can be lifesaving and there is certainly a time and a place for them, but personally, I think they're handed out too frequently. Antibiotics are really good at what they do, which is killing bacteria. What most people don't realize or consider is that they don't discriminate between good and bad bacteria—they wipe 'em *all* out. This is why, when our clients do need to take an antibiotic for a specific reason, I strongly recommend replenishing the good gut bacteria by taking extra amounts of a probiotic during the course of (and for an extended amount of time after finishing) their antibiotic treatment. Keeping your gut balanced is key!

Food Quality

Food quality is also an important factor. As mentioned, antibiotics can cause damage to your gut health, and unfortunately, many meat and dairy products are farmed with high doses of antibiotics. If the cow you're eating was given antibiotics, you're now consuming those antibiotics as well. Antibiotics found in conventional meat and dairy can cause inflammation. Look for grass-fed, organic meats that are free from added hormones and antibiotics and free-range chicken and turkey.

Likewise, when it comes to seafood, buy wild-caught fish to ensure you're not consuming heavy loads of chemical residue. It's important to remember that whatever your food was eating, you are also eating (think about cows given feed covered in pesticides or farm-raised fish that are fed exclusively genetically modified soy). Go for organic veggies and fruits—at least for the ones where you eat the outside skin. Also, choose real, whole fats, like butter, avocado, and unrefined coconut oil and ditch the more processed ones like vegetable oil, canola oil, sunflower oil and cottonseed oil.

Supplement Quality

Supplement quality is critical because most of the supplements out there contain ingredients that can be harmful and damage the lining of your gut, therefore promoting inflammation...even ones that claim to do the opposite and heal it! You're better off not taking any supplements at all than taking ones that can be provoking damage. At the same time, quality ones can boost your metabolism and weight loss by healing inflammation. We'll dive deeper into this in an upcoming chapter.

Stress

Because your gut is intricately linked to your state of mind (remember it's your "second brain"), stress affects your gut health and can wreak havoc on it. Stress management is also a crucial factor, so I will elaborate on this more later, too. For now, do your body a favor and stay rested, and practice stress management techniques so that it can focus on healing.

Exercise Smarter

Exercise can be beneficial, but we now know it's not the be-all, end-all when it comes to weight loss. It can actually stand in the way of you reaching your goals if you're doing too much of it and not giving your body a chance to rest. One of the reasons for this is because exercise produces an inflammatory response, which is one of the main reasons I decided to stop marathon running. Workouts make you weaker because they tear down your muscles. You only get stronger during recovery.

So how much is too much? It's different for everyone, and in general, I recommend exercising hard a few days a week and including rest days in between. You can bet that if you're doing too much of it and not giving your body a chance to rest, the physical stress you're putting on yourself won't be doing you any favors when it comes to your weight. This is why you see people who are exercising more than anyone on the planet, yet they aren't shedding a pound. Again, more on that to come...

Food Sensitivities and Allergies

The last way you can stop doing damage to your gut is by not letting food sensitivities and allergies go unchecked. Food sensitivities are at the root of many of our clients' difficulties with weight loss. If you have a food sensitivity or allergy and continue to consume the offending food, this will increase inflammation and cause damage to the intestinal tract.

This may sound obvious to some, but if you know you have a food allergy or sensitivity, completely avoiding the food is key to preventing further damage. Maybe you are lactose intolerant, meaning you don't have the enzyme to digest dairy, and you pop a pill when you are in the mood for ice cream since the pill is supposed to help lessen the damage. While the pill can mask the unpleasant symptoms associated with consuming the lactose your body can't tolerate, the damage is still being done. The symptoms are your body's own distress signal, its way of saying "SOS!" to let you know what's going on inside. We'll dive deeper into this topic in the next chapter.

That's how to *stop* the damage. Let's shift to step 2.

Step 2: Start Healing Existing Damage

The second step is to work on healing existing inflammation, leveraging anti-inflammatory foods and a few key supplements. Healing inflammation doesn't look the same for everyone, but these steps will get you on the right track.

First off, healthy fats—including saturated ones!— help heal inflammation. Translation: eat more butter, coconut oil, olive oil, olives, nuts, seeds and avocado (unless of course, you have sensitivities to any of those) as these are nourishing, healing fats. Just like some fats can be anti-inflammatory, certain fats can be pro-inflammatory. Be sure to choose healthy fats like the ones I listed and stay away from processed vegetable oils like canola, soybean, corn, cottonseed, rapeseed and sunflower oil. Good fats support many of the body's critical functions, including protecting against toxic overload, strengthening cell membranes (which make the skin more resistant to inflammation), stabilizing blood sugars, and providing a vehicle for your body to absorb fat soluble vitamins, leading to improved immune function. All of these properties help keep inflammation at bay, and support your weight loss goal.

Another great group of foods that help nourish the gut and reduce inflammation are fermented foods. Fermented foods are naturally high in favorable bacteria and that's how they support gut health and reduce inflammation. Fermented foods have gone through the process of fermentation which occurs when bacteria turns carbohydrates into lactic acid. This is a centuries-old technique that traditional cultures all over the world have practiced to increase the nutritive properties of a particular food, enhance flavors, and preserve their favorite produce and meat with the changing seasons. When we eat fermented foods, they replenish and diversify the bacteria in our gut. It's vital to have a healthy balance of good and bad bacteria in our gut to ensure overall well-being and weight loss, too. Sauerkraut, kimchi, kefir and kombucha are some healthy fermented foods. It's a good idea to try to include these in your eating regimen on a regular basis.

Along with consuming healthy fats and fermented foods, we find adding in healing supplements to your regimen provides the fastest, most effective results for getting on track with weight loss. Three key supplements that combat inflammation are: probiotics, L-glutamine, and fish oil. Together, the combination of these three supplements promote a healthy gut and proper digestion by rebuilding the intestinal lining, reducing inflammation, and restoring the good bacteria.

Probiotics are living microorganisms that are good, healthy bacteria. A probiotic supplement helps repopulate the healthy bacteria in the gut, which get depleted over time from eating inflammatory foods and taking antibiotics. A common misunderstanding is that probiotics are only for digestion and gut health. They are essential for the healing process and for weight loss. Newborn babies get their very first healthy bacteria in the form of bifidobacteria from breast milk, and it's important to make sure this isn't the only time our bodies are provided with it. For those of us who weren't breastfed, we never got that dose of good bacteria. Since the intestinal tract is regularly assaulted by stress, sickness, and environmental toxins, even if you're consuming fermented foods on a daily basis (which most of us aren't), everyone can benefit from supplementing with a probiotic at least once a day.

L-Glutamine is an amino acid that plays a vital role in rebuilding and maintaining the structural integrity of the thin lining of your digestive tract, which can become inflamed. It works with probiotics to promote good digestion and nutrient absorption while reducing inflammation and—bonus—it can ward off sugar cravings, too! L-Glutamine comes in capsule or powdered form, and I recommend using whichever works best for you. Many people, myself included, choose to use the powder in the kitchen and keep a bottle of capsules in their work bag or purse.

Finally, fish oil specifically targets inflammation and reduces it with the omega-3 fatty acids it provides. That's actually why a lot of our clients find relief in their back pain or joint pain when they start taking a high quality fish oil supplement. We can eat a lot of fish and still not get enough omega-3's to reduce inflammation at the rate we want to.

I put together a guide for you with my daily supplement recommendations for both men and women, along with the specific brands, doses and timing of when to take these. You can download that guide so that you can get started right away by visiting dietitiancassie.com/supplements.

Step 3: Be Patient and Consistent as Your Body Heals

Last but not least, know that patience and consistency are of utmost importance. Just like chronic inflammation didn't happen overnight, it doesn't heal overnight either. Give your body time to do its job and support it along the way. Changing habits, eating nourishing, real foods in balance, taking the key supplements, listening to your body, and giving it time to heal is imperative. Because chronic inflammation is the root cause of so many health issues including that stubborn weight loss, it's worth it to make the effort to reduce or eliminate the damage that is taking place in your body that you can't see.

If you were experiencing common symptoms associated with poor gut health and inflammation, it can be motivating to continue to do step #2, as you reap the benefits. Your energy levels may increase, your digestion could improve, maybe the constipation and diarrhea are gone or your sugar cravings have diminished. However, if you didn't have any of those symptoms before, it can be tougher to stick with it. This is where trusting the process becomes key. Know that if you haven't taken steps in the past to get your gut health up to par, then it probably *isn't* up to par. We have had clients who have focused on gut healing strategies and after two weeks, the stubborn pounds begin to just melt off. We've also seen it take several months. The amount of time completely depends on how much damage there is and how much healing needs to take place.

So, before you self-diagnose, and start to take action, how can you be sure that you actually have inflammation? Well, there isn't a single perfect test, but there are tests that, when paired with your symptoms, can give you an idea of the level of inflammation that exists in your body. Like I mentioned previously, nearly everyone today is living in a state of chronic inflammation unless they've taken measures to do something about it. Most of us have taken at least one round of antibiotics in our lifetime, or consumed processed, refined foods full of sugar and inflammatory oils. Whether intentionally or not, almost all of us have contributed to inflammation in our bodies. Since you picked up this book, I'm guessing you're experiencing at least one of the many symptoms of inflammation: weight loss frustrations. This is why I don't think testing is completely necessary, and at the same time, if you are interested in having some testing done, I'll provide you with these two good options:

1. C-Reactive Protein: CRP is a general blood marker of inflammation. It measures a protein that signals a

response to inflammation. It doesn't tell us the specific cause, but it does tell us that an inflammatory response exists. Make sure you don't have any acute inflammation going on (from a recent injury, sickness, or stubbed toe) when you get this test done because CRP will be elevated in response to any inflammation, acute or chronic. You want your CRP level well below 1 and preferably at 0, indicating that no inflammation exists.

2. Fasting Blood Insulin: A high insulin level when fasting may indicate chronic inflammation in the body. Remember, insulin will be higher as a response to elevated blood glucose because insulin acts as a vehicle for removing glucose from the blood and into storage. This test would be a second option, as the CRP test is usually our go-to for testing inflammation.

These two markers can be helpful, but we certainly don't consider them to be a comprehensive solution. I recommend following my anti-inflammatory PFC-balanced approach to nutrition and embracing the supplement regimen I outline in the guide at dietitiancassie.com/supplements to take care of any chronic inflammation that may exist—whether you know your test results or not. We can all benefit from reducing inflammation in our bodies on a daily basis.

By implementing these strategies, you can rebuild, repair, and support your gut, which in turn gives you more vitality and energy, and can help you lose weight. If you learn to listen to your body, give it time, and nourish it with good, healing nutrition, it will thank you by dropping the weight once it is ready. The first step is removing inflammatory triggers, the second is healing the damage with real food and natural supplementation, and the third is being patient and consistent to keep your body on the right track to lose weight.

CHAPTER EIGHT

FIGHTING THE SILENT FOOD FIGHT

Yogurt, skim milk, cereal, whole grain bread...What do they have in common? They are frequently touted as "health foods," but they could be standing in the way of your weight loss. Now, it's not your fault. Why would you ever think the foods you're consuming—the ones you were told were healthy—could be causing weight *gain*? You've probably been diligently including these in your daily meals and snacks. And, because you've been mislead by the media and the food industry alike, these foods may have been sabotaging you all along. You may not even know you're a victim. There's something you finally need to be taught, and it could be the key to unlocking that stubborn weight loss. It's a thing called food sensitivities.

Food sensitivities (not to be confused with food allergies—we'll touch on those in a bit) are a *disagreement* between a particular food and your body, resulting in inflammation and extra unwanted pounds. When it comes to food sensitivities, I've got a good news, bad news—well, momentarily "bad news" scenario. The good news is that if you identify that you have a food sensitivity, there is a very simple fix, and the results will be speedy. Okay, now for the "bad news." In order to get those results, you'll need to cut out all of the foods you could potentially be sensitive to from your diet in order to learn who the real culprit is. At first, it may seem a bit daunting to give up items that you perhaps have been enjoying. But, it can be done. When our clients decide to take action and cut out those foods from their diet, they are hesitant at first, but not for long. They quickly feel more energetic and engaged in life. Little did they know those foods were causing so much of their brain fog, lethargy, and—perhaps most exciting for them—those foods were causing their body to hold onto that stubborn fat. Once one or two offending items are removed, the weight starts to disappear.

Take Emily, for example. She's a successful working woman, a clinical nurse manager working in a hospital. She's educated and has it all together and under control...except for her weight. For fifteen years, Emily tried everything to lose weight. She was the stereotypical yo-yo dieter, dropping a few pounds here and there only to gain them back and then some. She would never actually get down to her desired weight. This was because she never got to the root cause of the weight gain to begin with. In addition to the weight problem, she also struggled with migraine headaches, feeling exhausted all the time, frequent diarrhea, and acne. Here's an interesting thing I will never forget about Emily: She overlooked telling me about all those issues for her first few appointments. Why? Was she embarrassed? Nope. It was because they had become her "normal." And so, she didn't even think twice.

When I told Emily that a food sensitivity was a very likely possibility—especially because a dairy sensitivity is a common cause of acne, the one symptom I could visibly see—she laughed and said there was no way that was the case; after all, she grew up on a dairy farm. The irony seemed too much. Unbeknownst to Emily at the time, it actually was the cause.

Food sensitivities are super tricky. Like Emily, you can count calories or grams or points or morsels all you want, but if day in and day out you are consuming a "wrong" food that your body can't tolerate, the numbers won't matter. You will continue to have an ongoing battle. You will not shed those stubborn pounds. This ties back to a topic we discussed earlier—inflammation. If you're sensitive to something, then *every time* you consume it, an inflammatory reaction takes place and your body has to fight it. Your body goes into "fight mode." It works hard to heal the areas that are damaged and inflamed from the offending food. That means if you're consuming the substance regularly, your body is constantly putting out fires and is chronically inflamed. Without knowing it, your body, in essence, is in a state of emergency. This is extremely draining and an inefficient use of your body's resources. When its energy is being consumed by battling something it doesn't agree with, the last thing your body is going to do is help you meet a weight loss goal.

Emily told me she had never been allergic to anything in her entire life. The thing is, you don't have to have an allergy to be sensitive to something. Food allergies are different than sensitivities. Allergies usually give an intense, more dramatic response. Food sensitivities are tricky because they're sneakier. It's typical to not *feel* a noticeable difference immediately after consuming a food you are sensitive to. We see clients all the time who drink a glass of milk and break out in acne a couple days later, not making the connection that the milk was the culprit. Or a sandwich at lunch causes a migraine headache in the evening. If you didn't have bread at dinner, why would you blame the slices from hours earlier? The reaction from a food sensitivity can happen a lot slower and is usually much more subtle than an allergy reaction. It can be trickier to identify and confusing because they don't show up on allergy tests. Emily's migraines, diarrhea, low energy and acne were more than enough red flags for my brain to jump to a food sensitivity—particularly dairy.

There are many other symptoms associated with food sensitivity. The common ones I've seen in clients include:

- Weight gain

- Skin problems, like acne, eczema, rosacea, rashes and dry skin

- Digestive issues, like gas, bloating, acid reflux, diarrhea, and constipation

- Migraine headaches

- Joint pain and muscle aches

- Low energy levels and fatigue

- Memory or concentration issues

Because they can take hours or even days to show themselves, it can be extremely helpful, maybe even critical, to track your symptoms. You can get my free symptom tracker at dietitiancassie.com/elimination. This allows you to make connections between what's happening in your body and what you ate. I don't expect you to remember what you ate three days ago—most of our clients can't remember what they had for breakfast!

A lot of the symptoms associated with food sensitivities are ones that we end up believing are our norm. Bloating, gas, headaches, weight gain, skin problems and low energy levels may be common, but not normal. There *is* a difference! These symptoms could be your body's way of expressing the inflammation that's happening as a result of eating foods it can't handle. Your body is trying to tell you something and maybe unknowingly, you blow it off or even try to mask the symptoms. And, you can be sensitive to a food, but that doesn't mean you were always sensitive to it. You could have developed a sensitivity after your gut health was compromised, leaving it too weakened to handle certain foods. When you heal the damage that's been done, you may find that you're able to tolerate them again.

I convinced Emily to ditch the dairy, even if it was just to humor me. At this point, she was so desperate to see even just a pound come off that she was willing to try anything. Within *days*, her acne began to clear up, her digestion improved, and her headaches vanished. Her email to me shouted that it was "too good to be true!" and "This is way easier than I thought it would be! I've been eating yogurt, cheese and drinking milk every day all my life and I thought it would be impossible to give them up, but not when I'm feeling this great!"

It didn't take long for the pounds to begin melting off. She lost five within the first week, and another five, and another five, until she was down fifty pounds. Emily continued to say it was too good to be true. I asked her several times if she missed dairy and she shook her head and said, "Not with the pounds coming off this easily. Now knowing the damage it was doing to my body, I can't believe I put it through that fight every day. No wonder I felt so awful. I can't believe weight loss can be this effortless."

When it came down to it, it wasn't about counting calories or exercising more. It was about taking away the inflammatory trigger that was standing in the way of Emily's weight loss. She could count calories or burn off calories all day long, but if the calories she was ingesting were from foods that her body couldn't handle, then it really didn't matter how many calories she was or wasn't consuming. We got to the root of the problem, and Emily is a different person now. Not only because she feels great at her goal weight, but also because she is forever done with the vicious cycle of dieting. For years, she put herself through a process where she felt cranky, foggy-brained, squeamish, and hardly energetic enough to make it through the day, especially on the days she was hit with a migraine. Identifying a food sensitivity, and keeping it out of her system, changed Emily's life. And Emily is certainly not the only client we've had experience this life-changing process.

The most effective way we've found to identify food sensitivities is through the process of elimination. This is the best way to determine how a certain food affects you. Allergy testing can be helpful, but I don't believe it is always the best answer, as many of the tests we have access to aren't completely accurate. It's perfectly normal for allergy tests to show false negatives, and they can be skewed based on whether or not you're eating certain foods. They also tend to overlook sensitivities. You can still have a sensitivity without having a full-blown allergy.

The top five most common foods people are sensitive to are gluten, dairy, eggs, soy and nuts. When you remove these foods and systematically bring them back into your lifestyle, it helps to decipher which foods are problematic and which are safe. Cut out the primary suspects for a few weeks (preferably six to twelve) before adding them back in. Remember, you've possibly been damaging your body daily with these foods, so you have to give it ample time to rest, recover and recalibrate. Then, pay attention to how your body reacts when you have or don't have that food in your daily eating regimen. When you eliminate the potential offending food for a period of time and then reintroduce it, your body will tell you what you need to know. If you don't have any problems when you add it back in for three days, then it likely isn't a food you are sensitive to. If you notice your symptoms return, then you know it's a food your body can't handle, at least for the time being. If you do find out you are sensitive to something, I recommend keeping it far, far away. Completely avoiding the food you're sensitive to is essential to preventing further damage. This doesn't mean you'll never be able to eat it again. You may be able to eat the foods that are causing you problems eventually, once your system has had a chance to heal. During the healing process though, you need to remove the inflammatory trigger completely to give your body a chance to recover. The key is to keep the food out of your system while you heal your body, and then you can try it again a few months down the road.

Now, some people question if it's a big deal to have a little bit of the food they're sensitive to in the future. I tend to tell them that, like Emily, most of our clients who discover a food has been harming their body and sucking the life out of them for too long, toss it out and never again let it return to haunt them.

You may experience such a radical change for the better that you don't even think twice about going back to the miserable way life used to be. Even having "a little bit" of a food you are sensitive to is likely to trigger the inflammatory process in your body and stand in the way of your success. Food sensitivities keep your body fighting and fired up every single day. Even if you've reached your weight loss goal before beginning to eat the offending food again, it will only be a matter of time before the pounds creep back on. It's not worth it. If you do get a craving for the food(s) you're sensitive to, remind yourself of your symptoms. Reflect on how long and frustrating a path it was to get here. Maybe you'll even smile as you acknowledge what a relief it is to finally understand what was happening in your body and feel empowered knowing what you know now. Knowledge is power.

For my free guide outlining our Elimination Diet Protocol and 7 days of PFC-balanced meal plans that we use with our clients as we help them through the process of identifying food sensitivities, go to dietitiancassie.com/elimination.

CHAPTER NINE

FINDING HARMONY IN YOUR HORMONES

Insulin, glucagon, ghrelin, leptin, estrogen, testosterone, cortisol—No, that's not a tongue twister. They're all hormones, and they're all critical pieces for your health! At the heart of it all, if your hormones are imbalanced, it's almost impossible for the pieces of your weight loss puzzle to come together. When your hormones are in harmony, your metabolism is supported and you feel amazing—you're energized, in control of your moods, your cravings fade away, and you're ready to conquer the world! On the flip side, when they're out of balance, you feel exhausted, out of control, and your metabolism tanks. *That* is when you gain weight.

Now, we've discussed a couple of important hormones already, like glucagon and insulin, and in upcoming chapters, we'll talk about other important hormones like cortisol, leptin, and ghrelin. Right now, I just want to talk about hormones in general. You see, you have a lot of hormones, and they all need to be in balance for you to get results. Hormones are like the thermostat of all of your body's functions. As they go up and down, they affect your moods, skin, hair, appetite, sex drive, metabolism, and—as is the primary purpose of this book—your ability to lose weight. On top of all that, hormones also affect *each other.*

You can think of insulin as your master hormone because when insulin is at work, the activities of other major hormones are suppressed. When insulin plays its trump card, all other hormones step out of the way. For this reason, keeping your blood sugar levels stable is vital, or else insulin takes over the show. Since, as you know, insulin's main job is to store fat, it's important to keep insulin's workload as light as possible. When insulin isn't working hard, you're not packing on more pounds.

There are a couple other hormone suspects that could be adding to your weight loss mystery. They are estrogen and testosterone. You probably know these as your female and male hormones, respectively. We all have both estrogen and testosterone in our bodies; it's just the ratios of one to the other that are different.

Estrogen is a hormone that is produced primarily in the ovaries in women and in the testes in men. A lot of people don't realize that estrogen dominance can occur in both men and women. Testosterone tends to be converted into estrogen when both men and women gain weight. Problems arise when estrogen levels are out of balance. This can easily happen when we are under stress, consuming processed foods, eating soy products, not sleeping enough, taking hormones (like the birth control pill), and even when we're exposed to estrogen-like compounds found in plastic and styrofoam. These problems continue to pile up if we aren't doing anything to eliminate the negative effects.

In women, when estrogen levels are too high, we see an increase in the prevalence of breast cancer, endometriosis, infertility and low libido. In men, excessive estrogen leads to an increased risk of prostate cancer, weight gain and low libido, as well. You need to have the right balance of estrogen and testosterone for your systems to be working properly and for you to ultimately shed pounds.

For women, hormones are always in flux. Our bodies are designed that way, for better or for worse. Our hormones change depending on where we are in our cycle and whether we have a cycle or not. Cravings, moodiness, fatigue, acne breakouts, bloating, insomnia, and uncontrollable emotions are common issues women face during puberty, pregnancy, their menstrual cycle, and menopause. The ebb and flow of the female body's delicate and natural hormone rhythms influence all aspects of physical and emotional wellbeing.

Many people aren't aware of this, but we really do have an incredible amount of control over our hormonal balance. Often times we brush off the negative side effects we're experiencing as a result of hormone imbalance, assuming it's just something we have to deal with. That's just the way it is, right?... It's not! There are ways to balance your hormones without hormone replacement therapy.

Benefits of Hormone Balancing

"I would have never thought that changing my nutrition would be what finally cured my weight gain...AND help me get pregnant!"

Kelsey found herself in my office seeking answers for the weight she'd put on over the last few years. However, it was what else she discovered during our work together that really changed her life. You see, she and her husband had been struggling with infertility for a while. She never guessed meeting with a dietitian would be what finally put her on the path to starting a family on top of shedding those stubborn pounds once and for all!

I took Kelsey on a hormone balancing adventure following the suggestions I'm about to outline for you that resulted in the weight loss she desired, among other bonuses like reduced cravings, disappearing headaches, and a baby! All through changes in her diet and a few supplements. Nothing else.

Here's a common scenario: Your doctor tests your hormone levels, some of them come back low, so he or she gives you a prescription for synthetic hormones to bring those levels back up. Synthetic hormones are fake and mimic the ones your body naturally produces.

There are a couple problems with this. The first is called a negative feedback loop. When you take hormones, your body, in turn, produces less. So, you never really get to the bottom of what cause the hormonal balance in the first place. Additionally, you end up suppressing your body's natural hormonal production.

So, How Does This Tie Into Weight Loss?

Hormone resistance is like the analogy we used earlier when discussing insulin resistance. Compare it to being in a noisy room—when you walk in, it's loud and you can't hear anything, but after a while, you get used to it. When this happens with your hormone receptors, they start to tune out the extra hormones that are being injected into your body, similar to how you cells tune out insulin and stop responding as they get worn out. This means more hormones circulating in your body, and the more of those, the harder it becomes to lose weight.

There are a few ways you can support your body's delicate hormonal balance through your nutrition and lifestyle before you take any synthetic hormones that might just exacerbate your problems.

Earlier, we discussed the importance of healthy fats and cholesterol and their role in keeping inflammation down. Another important role they both play is kick-starting the production of your hormones. Cholesterol and healthy fats are building blocks for your hormones, and, after having followed a low-fat diet, your hormones struggle to exist. Your liver has to work harder to produce cholesterol since you aren't getting it from your food. While it's true your body has an amazing ability to compensate when needed, when your liver has to continually focus on producing cholesterol to maintain balance, not only do you feel tired and out of whack, but your fat-burning is put on the back burner. Do your hormones a favor and choose healthy fats like coconut oil, olive oil and real butter, along with foods with cholesterol like shrimp, red meat, cheese, and eggs (including the yolks!). Stay away from the inflammatory fats like vegetable oil, soybean oil, peanut oil, and margarine.

▶ **Skip Soy!**

Avoiding foods with estrogenic properties like soy is also a great step towards supporting hormonal balance. Soy can negatively affect your hormones, and it's the root cause of the dreaded "man boobs."

▶ **Skip Stress!**

Avoid stress when possible. Stress is the enemy of a balanced hormonal system. In an upcoming chapter, we're going to talk about how stress plays a significant role in hormonal balance and your weight (as well as nearly every other area of your health). In short, when your body is stressed, it focuses on making cortisol, your stress hormone, and it takes a break from working on your other hormones. (That explains why you might notice a low sex drive when you're stressed out.)

Skip over-exercising! Take a break from the gym. I'll dive into other reasons why cutting back on your exercise regimen and stepping away from the gym can benefit your waistline. For the purpose of this chapter, you should know that too much exercise can wreak havoc on your hormones, too. (Which in turn can block your weight loss...remember, it's all connected!)

▶ **DON'T Skip Supplementation!**

The next step may be the most important one when it comes to hormones and your weight loss. You *must* keep your estrogen levels balanced—a task most easily done through key supplementation. This was one of the simplest additions to the hormone balancing adventure I took Kelsey on. For many people, this is the key to unlocking that stubborn weight loss, especially if it's something never focused on before. I created a free guide for you in which I outline two simple ways you can do this. Find it at dietitiancassie.com/hormones.

Lastly, hormonal balance can also impair the function of the gland that really controls your weight loss, which leads us to the next chapter.

CHAPTER TEN

THE GLAND THAT REALLY DICTATES YOUR WEIGHT LOSS

"My thyroid is normal," she stated confidently. "My doctor tested it and said it was normal, so we've ruled that out."

Jennifer felt she had done everything she could and still she found herself stuck, unable to get rid of those excess pounds—and now here sitting in my office. Of course, her weight wasn't the only struggle she had. I quickly learned she was tired all the time even though she was sleeping well. She was practically falling asleep at her desk job; she had frequent headaches, constipation, low energy levels, low libido, and hadn't had her period in several years. As she rattled the symptoms off to me, she kept coming back to her weight, as that was her biggest concern. She had been determined to get to the root of her stubborn weight loss on her own, which led her to read, research, and request testing of her thyroid. She had all the signs of low thyroid function, but the test came back negative.

Frankly, I was impressed with her determination, and also that she'd already learned the importance of the thyroid—such a common reason why people, especially women, are unable to shed the pounds. Yet, for some reason, it's something that's not really talked about, at least not nearly enough, which is why it is so frequently overlooked. Different studies have shown as many as 1 in every 8 females has an underactive thyroid! This is confirmed by the hundreds of clients I've seen struggling with it—many of whom don't know they are struggling because, just like Jennifer, when they have it tested, their lab numbers come back in the "normal range." I wasn't surprised to hear that her doctor said her thyroid function was normal after running a test. That wasn't enough for me to rule it out.

"Do you know your numbers?" I asked her.

"No, he just said it was normal," she replied. "I'm a mystery case. Good luck figuring me out." A smile finally crossed her face.

I smiled too, and simply replied, "No one's stumped me yet! I have no doubt—we'll get to the root of your stubborn weight loss, too."

Now, my confidence wasn't unwarranted. This conversation was not an uncommon one. When someone is exhibiting "mystery symptoms" while telling me their thyroid function is "normal"—well that's exactly where I like to start.

Master of Your Metabolism

Let's back up for a second. The thyroid isn't commonly understood. In fact, most people probably couldn't even point to where it's roughly located in the body (it is a butterfly-shaped gland centered in the back of your neck). That said, it's got a pretty big responsibility: it's the master of your metabolism! It's like the engine of a car; if it's not working well, then neither is the car. Likewise, when your thyroid isn't operating as it should, your metabolism isn't revved up and your whole body suffers, including your weight. Making sure your thyroid is in working order will do you a world of good, both for your energy levels *and* weight loss.

After I explained all of this to Jennifer, she asked the logical question, "It makes sense, but why would my numbers come back normal then?"

"A fair question," I said. "Things get interesting when it comes to the thyroid. Typically, we see most doctors covering up medical issues with everything from pills to potions—all without getting to the root cause of the problem. When it comes to thyroid function, however, I've noticed something different. Doctors will typically run a single TSH test, and if your number comes back in what is considered their "normal" range, they call it good and send you on your way."

"Now, there are a few problems with that. First of all, when it comes to your labs being "normal," it's important to note the ranges your doctor uses are based on a statistical average, which is created using people who go to the doctor, not healthy people. This means people with hypothyroidism are included in these reference ranges, so they don't hold a lot of weight in my book."

"Secondly, TSH is the main test practitioners use to determine thyroid function, and while it can be helpful, it in and of itself is quite limiting. Yet most doctors are *only* running this test. A TSH test works "backwards" in a sense. Your pituitary gland is your thyroid's CEO. It makes and secretes TSH (thyroid stimulating hormone) to tell your thyroid to work harder. So, if your TSH is elevated at all, it's a pretty good sign that your thyroid isn't working well. While the "normal" reference ranges that most doctors use are continually going down, most still consider a 2.5 or 3 to be "normal." To me, that's crazy, because why would your pituitary gland tell your thyroid to work harder at all if it's functioning normally? It wouldn't! I look for a TSH number to be as close to zero as possible, and consider anything above 0.3 to be a red flag for hypothyroidism."

"So, that's actually been the case with a lot of clients. The one TSH test is done, it comes back "normal," and they are sent on their way. In reality, their thyroid isn't working well enough for them to have the energy they need and to experience the weight loss they desire. It's absolutely possible to have abnormal thyroid function and a "normal" TSH level."

"Besides, it's not the only test we should be looking at. I recommend going well beyond the TSH test and getting a full comprehensive thyroid panel, including not just TSH, but also Free T4, Free T3, Reverse T3, Thyroid Peroxidase Antibodies (TPOAb) and Thyroglobulin Antibodies (TgAb). Now, you don't have to remember all those as it's rather complex. Don't feel bad if you're not comprehending what they are or the results they will give you! That's why I recommend meeting with a healthcare professional who specializes in functional medicine, preferably one with experience in thyroid conditions. All of these tests are important because they give you more specific information about your thyroid and where the issue may lie. They can tell you if it's having trouble producing thyroid hormones, converting them, attacking itself, et cetera."

Jennifer nodded and confirmed she hadn't heard anything about this before. That's a big part of the problem.

You see, the way conventional doctors are approaching the thyroid is leaving too many people undiagnosed. That said, even if they do end up diagnosing someone with an underactive thyroid, they'll either prescribe a thyroid replacement hormone, or they'll do absolutely nothing! The good thing is this is actually preferable on our end, because then we can take the time to address the real problem without having to counteract the side effects of a medication. For those who are already on a medication, I've actually had many clients who were able to reduce their dose, and even come off of it, after working with me for several months—all with the guidance of their medical doctor, of course.

Alright, a little more about the thyroid: I mentioned that it's a gland, and glands produce and secrete hormones to keep your body functioning properly. The two most important thyroid hormones are thyroxine (T4) and triiodothyronine (T3). T4 is the inactive form of thyroid hormone that's converted into T3—the active hormone that affects metabolism, and in turn, your weight. All of this needs to be working properly for you to have energy and lose weight. You can have lots of T4 hanging out, but if it's not being converted to T3, then your metabolism is in the tank. It's important to know all of your numbers to determine if your thyroid is working properly.

So, Why Might it Not Be Working Well?

There are a variety of factors that can disrupt your thyroid function, but before you can address the cause, you need to know what to look for. Signs of impaired thyroid function can include weight gain, hair loss (especially eyebrow hair), chronic fatigue (even with good sleep), swollen eyelids, a puffy face, frequent sickness, mood swings, mental fog, anxiety, irregular periods, cold hands and feet, constipation, dry skin, hair and nails, and low libido—these are all symptoms of hypothyroidism.

Jennifer had many of the signs of impaired thyroid function, and until we addressed her thyroid, she wasn't going to be able to reach her weight loss goal, not to mention get rid of all of her other symptoms that I would argue were just as dangerous as her weight.

Since I'm a detective dietitian, I like to investigate and figure out what's really going on, instead of just recommending something (such as a medication) to cover up the symptoms. Impaired gut health, nutritional imbalance, chronic inflammation, stress, strenuous endurance exercise, food sensitivities, hormonal imbalance, radiation, zinc deficiency, alcohol, hormonal changes and/or soy consumption could be all culprits in diminishing your thyroid's effectiveness. Like I told Jennifer at that first meeting, it's a complex topic and as you may have noticed already, a lot of things are related (and you probably recognize a lot of these culprits from previous chapters in this book)!

Even if your lab data comes back "normal," I recommend a simple DIY test you can do at home that can give you an idea of how well your thyroid is working (or not working). Get an old school (mercury) thermometer and take your basal temperature (under your arm) right when you wake up for five consecutive mornings. If the average of five morning readings is below 97.6 ° F, this can be an indication that you have impaired thyroid function since low body temperature is correlated with low thyroid function.

There are many things you can do to support your thyroid. I'll outline a few here, and you can find the rest in my thorough guide to supporting your thyroid at dietitiancassie.com/thyroid.

▶ Eat PFC-balanced!

s outlined in Chapter One—this is really important when it comes to supporting your thyroid. Impaired thyroid function can cause inflammation, which can take over your body and inhibit the conversion of T4 to T3. This makes your cells less responsive to thyroid hormones. Eating in PFC-balance keeps your blood sugar levels stable which prevents further inflammation from occurring, and inflammation can block your thyroid from working properly. It's a vicious cycle. The combination of protein, at least 2 tablespoons of healthy fats, and nutrient-dense carbohydrates at every single meal and snack helps to calm inflammation, thereby keeping your thyroid in check.

▶ **Eat Enough Carbs**

When it comes to thyroid function, it's important to be sure you're getting in an adequate amount of carbohydrates. Not eating enough carbohydrates can impair thyroid function since insulin is required for the conversion of T4 to T3, and insulin levels will be low if you aren't eating enough carbs. Because of this, I still recommend carbohydrates mainly from vegetables, but I suggest making sure a few of your carbohydrate servings are starchy veggies or fruit every day. The protein is also of particular importance because it contains an amino acid called tyrosine, which helps support your thyroid by encouraging the production of thyroid hormones.

▶ **Avoid Gluten!**

This is important for a variety of reasons (many of which we've covered already), and in this case, it's especially important for thyroid support. The link between gluten and thyroid dysfunction is that the composition of thyroid hormone receptors are very similar to gluten. If the body thinks gluten is a toxin, it can confuse the thyroid for a toxin, thus producing antibodies that cause it to attack itself. If you follow my recommended eating plan, PFC is naturally gluten free.

▶ **Skip Soy!**

Soy can negatively affect your thyroid because the isoflavones in soy interfere with production of T3 and T4, which is necessary for a well-functioning thyroid. I've also come to the conclusion that soy can lead to hypothyroidism, based on my experience working with clients with low thyroid function. Regardless, it's just not worth consuming soy, especially since soy can also cause a host of other problems for your health.

▶ **Heal Your Gut!**

Poor gut health can contribute to thyroid disease, and thyroid hormone dysfunction can wreak havoc on your gut health, too. The gut health recommendations in Chapter Eight are the ones I recommend for anyone suspecting impaired thyroid function.

▶ **Manage Stress!**

Stress is a significant offender of the thyroid. High stress levels will produce excess cortisol, which can inhibit thyroid stimulating hormone (TSH) and T4 and lead to inflammation, which in turn wreaks havoc on thyroid health. You can find healthy ways to manage stress in your life in an upcoming chapter.

▶ **Lastly, Check for Food Sensitivities, Intolerances, and Allergies.**

I'm only going to retouch on this briefly, as we just spent a whole chapter on it, but it's important so know this: a thyroid imbalance can cause food sensitivities, and conversely, consuming foods your body is sensitive to can contribute to impaired thyroid function because of the inflammatory response it triggers. Sadly, it's a two way street. If you have a sensitivity, allergy, or intolerance, your body will spend its energy fighting the offending food item. This makes your thyroid work overtime, which negatively affects the rest of your body—as you may very well know. Allergy testing isn't always the best answer, as many of the tests we have access to aren't very accurate. The best test is eliminating a food for at least 3-4 weeks (preferably 6-12), and then adding it back in while evaluating what happens to your body. If that doesn't do the trick, try working with a qualified dietitian coach who can help guide you in the process of pinpointing food sensitivities.

So again, I recommend starting with these steps. You can find the rest of my advice in my guide to supporting your thyroid at dietitiancassie.com/thyroid.

Curious to know how things turned out with Jennifer? Well, here's what happened once she implemented my thyroid support recommendations:

Just six weeks after we discussed my recommendations, she began changing. A lot. First, she had a dramatic improvement in energy, her constipation completely vanished, and she even started shedding a few of those stubborn pounds that she had no success with on her own for so long.

After twelve weeks, her period came back. That was a big deal because menstruating is a sign of healthy hormonal balance, a side effect of healthy female functioning, and it's a natural process that your body is supposed to go through.

So, if you've tried everything to lose weight, but haven't examined your thyroid function, this could very well be the (undiagnosed) key to unlocking that stubborn weight loss!

PART 3

KEY MAXIMIZERS: REMEMBER THESE S'S FOR FEWER "LBS"

CHAPTER ELEVEN

SUPPLEMENTS: THE SCARY TRUTH ABOUT WHAT'S INSIDE YOUR MEDICINE CABINET

"I'm doing everything I can to help my body shed the pounds!" Amanda said as she walked into her first appointment, proudly carrying a grocery bag overflowing with bottles of pills. Like many people on a quest for weight loss, Amanda was blindly taking everything in this bag, in the hopes of finding the magical combination to cure her of her weight issues.

As we sifted through the bottles together, Amanda was confronted with a difficult truth. Many of the supplements she was taking on a daily basis to help her lose weight could have actually been adding to her weight gain all along! Unbeknownst to her, some of the supplements listed harmful ingredients on the labels, like artificial sweeteners, refined oils, and other additives and fillers. When I realized that she was taking a lot of these supplements multiple times a day, those sweeteners, oils and additives were really adding up—especially around her waistline. The problem was that any one (or all!) of the supplements in her bag could have been in the way of her weight loss goal. Then there's the even more distressing news.

It's likely her supplements not only contained the harmful ingredients listed on the label, but there could be more, and it could be worse. Supplements are unregulated because they don't have to go through any FDA approval process. This means companies aren't required to list everything that's in the pills on the label. Who knows what all could have been in the ones in Amanda's grocery bag? This is what happens when regulation laws aren't in place. We know this is happening. It's been confirmed by several studies, including a shocking one in 2013 conducted by the New York State Attorney General's office, showing that 4 out of 5 supplements on the shelves of popular retailers contain NONE of the herbs or ingredients listed on the labels (Newmaster et al., 2013)! So, there is a mystery combination of unknown ingredients and additives in these products that we, as consumers, aren't even privy to. All of that junk is harmful for your body! It deadens metabolism, impairs your thinking, reduces immune function, increases inflammation, and generally causes more harm than good.

I had to break it to Amanda that her supplements were very likely what was preventing her from reaching her weight loss goal. Her disappointment was evident. "That said, replacing these with a few high quality supplements could be the key to unlocking your weight loss goal. Another plus is that you probably don't need to take even half as many supplements as you brought in today. The key is taking the right, high quality ones that actually work."

"But wait—" She said. "Ugh! What's up with supplements being full of harmful junk? You have *no* idea how much money I've spent on these things!"

"I know," I replied with a sigh. "It's heartbreaking, really. You aren't alone, either. We see this happening *all* the time with our clients and in the industry in general. When clients come to us, just like you have, they're often investing in these supplements in an attempt to improve their health, and those very supplements are what end up making them heavier and sicker than when they weren't taking any of them at all. You wouldn't think to blame your lack of weight loss on the supplements that are supposed to help you lose that weight, right? Well, that's often exactly the case."

You've got to be on the defense when it comes to what you're putting in your body. (Because trying to be healthy isn't hard enough, right?! Sheesh!) Just as it's important to be mindful of the food you put in your body, you need to be mindful about your supplement intake, too.

So, why aren't supplements regulated? That's a discussion for a whole different kind of book. Besides, regulation wouldn't solve everything anyway. The FDA regulates our food, yet a lot of fake, toxic foods still make it through the process and get a "pass" when in reality, they're barely even food. (Velveeta, anyone?)

There's a lot of confusion about supplements, and not just for Amanda. Even as a dietitian, I had to dig deep and get my hands really dirty to get to the bottom of all the confusion and nonsense that's out there. At first, I didn't think supplements even mattered. There was a long period of time when I thought people could just get their nutrients from food, and I didn't see the need for supplements. In fact, I didn't even give them a shot until I had hit rock bottom with my sugar addiction.

In dietitian school, I wasn't taught much about supplements. I certainly didn't know how harmful a supplement could be or how many scary, shady ones exist on store shelves that make their way into our cabinets. As a result, I didn't really know there was such a range of quality levels. I didn't realize how effective the high quality ones could be for just about every health concern anyone could ever deal with, including weight loss.

So, when it comes to supplement quality, I have good news and some bad news. The good news is that there *are* high quality, third-party tested supplements that are regulated and effective. Sadly, these supplements are hard to find since they don't exist on grocery store or drugstore shelves. They can only be found through licensed healthcare professionals. Even then, still not all supplements sold by healthcare professionals are quality. It's just as frustrating for me as it is for you.

After explaining all of this, I could see how discouraged Amanda was, so it was time to dive deeper into the good news.

"When you're taking high quality supplements, they can be extremely effective—not only at filling in nutrient gaps when you deviate from your healthy eating regimen—because I know no one is perfect!—but also in reducing inflammation, kicking sugar cravings, and shedding pounds. So, just like we see so many of our clients move further away from their goals by taking junky, unapproved supplements, we see the opposite happen when they take supplements that are third-party tested—ones that contain what they say they contain, ones that actually work. They tend to reach their weight loss goals even faster."

I shared with Amanda how this was something I was so personally frustrated with that I was determined to create a reliable solution. The supplements I was personally taking just weren't cutting it. They weren't fresh enough. I was sick of the questionable ingredients. I couldn't be picky about things like the fact that I prefer my glutamine capsules and multivitamins to be more potent so that I could take fewer of them, and how I don't want my vitamin D bathed in inflammatory refined soybean oil...the list goes on. That is why I finally took the initiative and created my own line of supplements, VeroVive™[3], that I have complete control over and meet all of my criteria. I did the research and the work so that you wouldn't have to worry about it.

It's important to me that my line of supplements is regulated by a third-party. So, they must be rigorously tested and monitored throughout the manufacturing process, both for their purity and the quantity of all dietary ingredients. That means waving goodbye to the frustration surrounding shady supplements and unethical labels. It means people like you don't have to anxiously stare at labels on the store shelves, trying to sort out the "good" from the mischievous supplements! VeroVive™ is regulated and made from only the finest ingredients. You never need to question the quality or wonder if they contain hidden junk, fillers, or sweeteners. Ever. You won't find a brand more focused on quality, purity, and potency—which means fewer pills, more nutrients, and better results—something we see every day with our clients. Whether you're the type of person who looks at every single label on every product, or you're like Amanda and you prefer not to have to think about that kind of stuff at all, you can trust the supplements I've created, and you don't have to be duped by supplements ever again.

I told Amanda that I recommend either taking high-quality pharmaceutical grade supplements that are regulated, like the VeroVive™ line or none at all. While it's a strong statement, it's

---

[3] VeroVive™ is Italian for perfect, complete life...and that's why we take supplements! We all want that perfect, complete life and that's what this line of supplements helps you achieve. rfvitamins.com/verovive

the truth. You can do a lot more harm than good by ingesting shady supplements filled with potentially harmful ingredients. That's why the products I recommend are only ones that are regulated, and I personally wouldn't take anything else.

The Need for Key Nutrients

I asked Amanda if she was willing to walk out to the dumpster with me to get rid of all those bottles of pills. I asked her if she was ready for a fresh start.

"Absolutely. My fresh start begins now. I guess I should have asked this a long time ago, but do I really need supplements to help with my weight loss goal?"

"It's a great question." I told her, "Supplements are that piece of the puzzle many people don't realize they're missing, and they can be that hidden key to unlocking your weight loss. No matter how hard we try, getting all of the nutrients we need from food alone is incredibly difficult. If you can get everything your body needs from real food to run most efficiently and lose the weight, that's great! Most of the time, though, eating healthy just isn't enough, especially with a hefty goal of weight loss. Even when we're eating "right," we likely aren't meeting our vitamin and mineral needs. Mineral depletion in the earth's soil, exposure to environmental toxins, and the effects of chronic stress are just a few of the many reasons for that. When you lack key nutrients, your body simply can't function as efficiently as it should. That's why you experience exhaustion, mood swings, sugar cravings and brain fog...and you just can't seem to shed those last five or fifty pounds—no matter how hard you try! It's way harder to lose weight when your nutritional needs aren't being met."

"Whether or not you choose to supplement also depends on how quickly you want results. It is possible to heal your body and get it in balance through real food, but that may not be enough, and it will definitely take way more time. For clients who choose to just stick with eating real food first, we often find after a few months they become frustrated because they're working so hard and not getting the more tangible results they want to see. They end up adding in supplements anyway, and really start noticing a difference."

"I find that most people who are coming to see me are already frustrated and ready to start seeing results *now*, so they generally take the high quality supplements to help expedite their results. It's up to you. Start with just eating real food first, and then add in supplements when you're ready, or you can hit the ground running and start with both to help you reach your goals faster. I recommend the latter. My guess is you're sick and tired of struggling with this and ready to get to the bottom of it so you can get on with your life, am I right?"

"Absolutely!" Amanda replied emphatically. "The sooner the better. So which supplements should I take?"

Because women and men have different biological needs, there are specific daily essentials—supplements everyone can benefit from taking on a daily basis—for each sex. These supplements serve as the foundation for your weight loss goal, and while you may choose to add in others, such as those I make mention of in other chapters of this book, the daily essentials are a critical starting point, no matter what other pieces of your puzzle may yet need to come together.

For Amanda, I went through each of the women's daily essentials, and I did that for you, too. I put together a guide with my daily recommendations for both men and women, along with the specific doses and timing of when to take these, and a special promotion for you as a reader of this book. You can download that guide so that you can get started right away. Just visit dietitiancassie.com/supplements.

Amanda went on to reach her weight loss goal, just months after ditching the bad supplements and embracing the good. Now that you have a better understanding about supplements and the potential havoc they've been playing on your body, it might be time to go into your medicine cabinet and dump all the "grocery store bought" brands that you can't trust, too. Again, it's better to take no supplements than to take the wrong ones. If you want to finally have supplements that you can trust in your cabinets, then download that guide at dietitiancassie.com/supplements for my best recommendations.

CHAPTER TWELVE

STRESS: HOW BALANCING YOUR LIFE CAN BALANCE THE SCALE

"If I had known taking a ten day vacation would be the answer to my weight loss problem, I'd have done it ten years ago!" Kim exclaimed.

With a high end job as the VP of marketing for a well-known firm in Philadelphia, she routinely worked between ten and twelve hour days, five to six days a week, never getting a break. The last thing she had time for was a vacation. Her frequent work travels were as close as she'd get. Kim confessed to me that it'd been years since she had even taken a vacation day. She couldn't remember exactly when the last time she took a day off was. She had too much work to do to cash them in. Heck, she didn't even take a day off on the weekend. The piles of work were too big to ignore. That very work ended up being the reason she gained so much weight.

Based on her work calendar, you'd wonder how on earth Kim had time to get to the gym four days a week, but she did. Her life revolved around the career grind and trying to be healthy. She knew more about GMOs, organic food, and biochemical processes than any other client I'd taken on. She was diligent about her exercise schedule, even when she worked late, and she spent her weekends meal prepping (when she wasn't working from home, that is). Yet, despite her best efforts and dedication to eating healthy and working out, she gained weight.

She was superwoman. And her waistline was paying for it.

How Stress Affects Weight

Kim worked with me for twelve whole months before taking that much-needed vacation. We had addressed a lot of things in the course of that year, and she had seen significant improvement in her headaches, her sleep, her moods, and even her sugar cravings, and in spite of all that, those stubborn pounds still weren't dropping.

We had touched on stress management several times, but it seemed like a race with no end in sight. She wasn't willing to cut back from her job and couldn't seem to find time for any stress management other than Friday night yoga.

"But, that's more than most people do anyway, right?" Kim asked me hopefully.

"It probably is." I responded. "However, most people are overweight."

I went on to explain, "Stress can sabotage all of your weight loss efforts, which is what I think you're experiencing. Your demanding lifestyle and career are putting more stress on your body than it was designed to handle. It's common and widely accepted to just brush it off—that's what most of us do. We live in a society where being stressed out is viewed as equivalent to being a productive, valuable, contributing citizen."

"Stress is a big deal. It affects all aspects of your health. Nearly every nutrient your body stores can be depleted by stress. It can significantly affect digestion and your gut health by suppressing stomach acid, weakening the gut lining, and harming good bacteria—thus compromising immunity. It affects your health and well-being in a number of ways."

Stress affects your metabolism and weight like a domino effect.

Take, for example, the hormone cortisol—possibly the most important hormone in your body because without it, you couldn't handle stress. Cortisol is known as your "stress hormone," since it's triggered in response to stress. Cortisol regulates your "fight or flight" response, and it exists as a survival mechanism. It is triggered when you are in danger. It is meant to be released in small doses and for short lengths of time. It serves its purpose when you need to kick into high gear by increasing your blood sugars and blood pressure. You can thank cortisol for the surge of energy you get when you are being chased by a tiger.

Thanks cortisol! You saved our lives while we were in the Sahara! Oh...wait. We don't live in the jungle anymore. Well, perhaps we do, but now it's a concrete jungle. That cortisol isn't being release on the rare occasion when a predatory animal is in our midst. Now, it's being released like a steady IV drip while we dodge bad drivers during rush hour, before we give our weekly staff presentation, while we listen to our boss give us our quarterly review, while we listen to the teachers say our children are falling behind in class, while we watch the 6 o'clock news and hear about some new thing in the world that is out to kill us....Our bodies weren't designed for this kind survival mode on steroids.

So, How Does This Tie into Your Waistline?

"Like I said, cortisol causes your blood sugars to rise. That means any time you are stressed out, you have elevated blood sugars, which is as if you're eating high amounts of sugary foods all day long. As you know, this causes insulin—your fat storing hormone—to come out to do its job of transporting sugar from your bloodstream to your cells to be stored as fat. And, well, you see where that can lead. This is how you gain weight when you're stressed...independent of your nutrition...without even eating any more, less, or differently!"

"To make matters worse, insulin tends to overcompensate, which means once it's done its job, your blood sugar levels drop below normal. What do you crave when you have low blood sugar? More sugar! The spikes and crashes in blood sugars take us for a ride on the blood sugar roller coaster, which can lead to a vicious cycle of weight gain with sugar and carb cravings. Simply having extra cortisol present will increase your appetite, particularly for sugar and carbs, because cortisol wants to replenish your body's stores that it used fighting against or running from the stressful thing that you're dealing with. That helps to explain why people who are stressed tend to grab sugary foods as a stress reliever, too."

Levels of Stress

Next, let me distinguish between the two levels of stress. This conversation may sound familiar because, just like there are two kinds of inflammation, acute and chronic, there are two kinds of stress. There's acute stress and chronic stress—both of which cause your adrenal glands to kick out cortisol.

Acute stress is short-lived and associated with everyday stressors. We're genetically wired to deal with acute stress in small, brief amounts; however, it becomes a problem when it persists. Acute stress could be a result of meeting a deadline, or getting cut off in traffic, or worrying about being late for an appointment, or lack of sleep. Symptoms of acute stress may include anxiety, headaches, shortness of breath, heart palpitations, and/or muscle pain.

The second level of stress is the most concerning, and this is what Kim had been dealing with.

"You're living in a "fight or flight" state of stress all day long. And, you aren't alone. Chronic stress is the type that many of us are dealing with on an ongoing basis. When all those small stressors continue piling up and we fail to manage them, chronic stress develops. This type of stress wears us down. Many people, like you, have been dealing with chronic stress for years, which is incredibly detrimental to our health. Cortisol is stressful on your body, and it wasn't designed for this type of stress. Because of that, when you're chronically stressed out, inflammation ensues."

Kim was taking it all in. I could see her making the connections with a heavy nod of her head.

"When you're experiencing chronic stress, it's bound to result in chronic inflammation. That inflammation damages healthy tissue in your body. This is scary because the symptoms aren't obvious, and it manifests itself in different ways from one person to another. It can present itself in a variety of ways, like migraine headaches, heart disease, and weight gain. Your body sees it as a fire, and it's always going to prioritize taking care of the inflammation before anything else. This means that it's going to be really tough for your body to lose weight, without first reducing inflammation. Since inflammation is the root cause of weight gain, and of course, chronic disease, it's vital to manage our stress levels to prevent this damaging buildup and to help you shed those unwanted pounds." I could tell Kim knew where I was going with this, but that didn't stop me.

"Stress sets the stage for inflammation and slows down metabolism by spiking cortisol levels and driving the insulin response. Being stressed day in and day out like you are means you're never giving your body a break. You're living with that tiger chasing you all the time. The more stressed you are, the worse your ability to deal with stress becomes, making it a vicious cycle."

Kim sat back in her seat. "Okay, so my job is this tiger that's been chasing me for years, and even though I'm doing all of this running, I won't be able to lose weight until I lose the tiger? What am I supposed to do? Quit my job?" She ended on an exasperated note.

I told her, "Well, not necessarily, no. The good news is that you have the power to manage your stress." I paused and looked her in the eyes. "Look, this topic hits close to home for me, too. I'm a hard worker and an overachiever at times, just like you, so I'm continually trying to achieve balance in my life and implement ways to reduce my stress and mitigate its harmful effects. The reality is that if we're not doing forms of regular stress management, then all of our best efforts with nutrition, exercise, sleep, supplements—*all of it*—is sabotaged. Now, your Friday night candlelit yoga is a great start. What else could you do?"

For the rest of her session, Kim and I brainstormed ways she could manage her stress (without quitting her job). I've compiled the results of our brainstorming (in addition to a few other ideas of my own) in a free guide for you to download at dietitiancassie.com/stress. I'm sharing these with you in hopes that they'll inspire you to find strategies that work for you so that you can feel at ease and find peace and balance, even during the most hectic of times.

As we were wrapping up, I could see Kim have a light bulb moment. She laughed and said, "Well, what I really need is a vacation!" Whether or not she had meant it jokingly, I held Kim accountable to that. While it took a few months to unfold, that's exactly what Kim did.

It was fun to see a completely different side of Kim, both as we kept in touch about her vacation plans and, of course, upon her return. Her all-or-nothing personality was sometimes tricky to work with considering our balanced approach, but it wound up being helpful once I really got her onboard with this vacation! Kim went all out and planned a 10-day vacation at a beach resort on Anna Maria Island in the Gulf of Mexico—the perfect getaway.

I was even able to convince her to keep her cell phone on airplane mode once she arrived at her destination. It took a few arrangements for this happen, like making it very clear at her workplace that she would not be responding to any emails and making sure her family and friends had an emergency number should they need to reach her, but she said it was so worth it. She didn't know that she could do it. It had been ages since she'd completely disconnected. Not only did she mentally need a vacation, but her body did, too.

Kim returned from her vacation not only the most cheerful I've ever seen her, but also ten pounds lighter.

"A miracle!" she exclaimed in a chipper, child-like voice. "It's not like I went to a healthy eating resort...I allowed myself to have delicious food and even some drinks, and the only exercise I did was a couple long walks on the beach. I've been working so hard to lose the weight, and a *vacation* ended up being what I needed in a million and one ways!"

Taking that vacation was a big answer to Kim's weight loss, and if stress is the key to unlocking her stubborn weight loss, it very well be could be a turning point for you, too. While a vacation can be the perfect way to reset, hopping on a plane to paradise isn't the only option. This is why it's important to include daily stress management strategies in your life, since we can't be on vacation every day anyway.

Daily Stress Busters

There are a few specific things I do during stressful times, and upon Kim's return, we discussed these and she vowed to practice them, too.

While we know the importance of eating well, it's especially important to make PFC-balanced eating an even greater priority during stressful times. When we're stressed out, it can be easy to put nutrition on the back burner and even give ourselves permission to eat processed, sugar-loaded snacks to "help" us through the stress. Kim wasn't overly prone to this, but a lot of us are. I know myself well enough to know that if I allow myself to dabble in the sugar realm, then I'll slip into the blood sugar roller coaster, and, as you know, that ride will only add more stress to your body. Be sure you're eating enough, too. If you undereat, your brain will panic and release cortisol which will compound your stress! We feel more balanced, stable, and able to make better decisions amidst stressful times when we're fueling our bodies with PFC every 3-4 hours. Eating this way prevents your blood sugar from spiking and crashing on that dreaded blood sugar roller coaster.

Make sure you build in some "me" time. Even if it's only five minutes a day; hopefully, some days you are able to set aside more than that. Five minutes every day is better than thirty-five minutes once a week. It's important to have time to think, process, and meditate or pray—every day, and especially during stressful times. This will help you feel centered and offer perspective into the things that matter and the things that really don't matter as much (after all, when we're stressed, even the littlest things can seem like the biggest deal). Personally, I make this a top priority, because if I just "pencil" it in, I know something will inevitably override it, so I have to be sure to block off time in my schedule for it. For me, this usually ends up being first thing in the morning. You know your schedule best, so fit it in where you can.

Stress support supplementation works wonders. In fact, this is one of the supplement categories my team and I are most frequently asked about. It's smart to give extra support for your body through stressful times. Your body will work better for you when you help negate the effects of stress with the nutrients it needs to push through these times. I've found the times when I am stressed are truly when it's most beneficial for me to supplement. Stress sucks the nutrients out of your body. So, by giving your body added supplementation, you counteract those damaging effects by promoting nutrient absorption (which stress depletes) and reducing some of that inflammation (which stress causes). I outline the supplements I take and recommend for stress support in the guide I created for you at dietitiancassie.com/stress.

My next suggestion is say no. Learning how to say no is a skill. Most of us have too much on our plates (so to speak), and that's the very reason why we're stressed. It's stressful being non-stop on the go, so determine what's really important to you, and what you can do to clear up your schedule. Saying "no" may seem like a simple solution, and I understand it isn't always as easy as it sounds, but it is a powerful, straightforward way to take control of your time and energy. Take out a journal and list your priorities and the things you *need* to do and the things that would be *nice* to do. Then prioritize the things that would be nice to do, and as these opportunities arise, begin to cut out the ones that just might cause you stress.

Lastly, make sure you talk about your stress. It's important to get things off your chest! Talk to a friend, a counselor, or a dietitian coach, and let it all out! It feels so good and it's so good for you. If you don't feel comfortable sharing with a friend or family member (especially if they are causing the stress!), another option is to check out our PFC Club Membership Community at dietitiancassie.com/community. Many of our members have found comfort and community in like-minded individuals who are on a similar journey to a healthy lifestyle. Meeting with a dietitian coach is also a great way to vent to somebody who isn't only a good listener, but can also provide individualized, evidence-based recommendations on other ways to deal with stress. Our clients tell us they look forward to their sessions so much because they know they can reveal their real selves and struggles without worrying about being judged or shamed. You can always count on us for supports. Afterall, we know that overall health is about more than just what we eat!

So if you're trying to cope with chronic stress right now, and it's starting to affect your body and weight in some of the ways I've outlined, why don't you go download my free guide for even more stress management tips? Then you can reap the benefits of unlocking one more key to that stubborn weight loss! Get your guide at dietitiancassie.com/stress.

CHAPTER THIRTEEN

SLEEP: WHAT YOU DO IN BED MATTERS TO YOUR WAISTLINE

Lori was really in the groove with her PFC-balanced eating and pretty much all of the other areas I've covered so far. She lost ten pounds in just three months, which she was thankful for and excited about. However, then her weight loss stalled in the last month. It was a mystery we were determined to solve.

"How are you sleeping at night?" I asked her. When she started her coaching with me, she'd been sleeping eight hours a night, but we hadn't touched on sleep for a while. Knowing how crucial a role it plays in weight loss, I decided it might be time to check back in.

"Fine, I think. I don't wake up to go to the bathroom or anything."

"What time do you go to bed and wake up in the morning?" I asked.

Lori thought about it and said, "Well, I'm usually in bed by nine—9:30 at the latest, and I wake up between 6:30 and 7:00 based on when my sleep app wakes me up."

Nine and a half hours, I thought. "How do you feel when you wake up?" I asked her.

"Absolutely exhausted." she replied.

There it was. That was it. Despite the fact that she was in her bed for nine plus hours, she was sleeping like crap. No wonder she hit a weight loss stall. All systems need to be working properly for your body to lose weight, and sleep plays a critical role in that.

Sleep controls the hormones leptin and ghrelin, which control our appetite and have an effect on the fat-burning and storing hormones, glucagon and insulin, which we covered earlier. Lack of sleep can increase cortisol, that stress hormone we discussed in the last chapter, causing your blood sugar levels to rise and your pancreas to secrete insulin. That insulin stores the sugar you eat as fat, resulting in weight gain. Both the *quality* and *quantity* of your sleep matter when it comes to losing weight. I told Lori it would be imperative to make sleep her next top priority.

"Actually," Lori said, "about that sleep app you told me to download…I did that, and I've been tracking the quality and quantity of my sleep." I was happy to hear that. Since it's not just the time they "clock in" to their bed that counts, but the quality of their sleep that matters (much like our approach to calories, yes?!), we encourage our clients to become aware of their sleep quality. This app I recommended for Lori encourages awareness as it's able to monitor and report on how much of your time in bed was actually spent getting quality sleep (I tell you more about it in the sleep hygiene guide I put together for you at dietitiancassie.com/sleep). She went on to say, "I found it peculiar that it says my sleep quality is poor, even though I don't wake up at night."

"I'm glad you mentioned that," I said. "Even though you may not realize you're not sleeping soundly, you still aren't. That's affirmed not only by what your app is telling us, but also the fact that you're exhausted despite being in bed for over nine hours every night."

I told Lori when she doesn't get enough sleep, she's facing bigger concerns than just fatigue or moodiness. I explained how her lack of sleep was affecting her hormones and how it was standing in the way of her weight loss goal.

As I mentioned, leptin and ghrelin are two hormones that are big players in regulating appetite. Leptin is your satiety or "I'm full" hormone, and it is secreted in fat cells to tell you to put your fork down—it decreases appetite. Ghrelin, your hunger hormone, is secreted in the lining of your stomach when it's empty, and increases appetite. When ghrelin increases, so does your appetite, specifically your appetite for sugar and carbs. Not snoozing enough lowers levels of leptin and increases ghrelin which stimulates your appetite. When there's an increase in ghrelin, up go your appetite and sugar cravings. This also means you still feel hungry after you eat. Besides, who hasn't reached for a mocha, bag of chips, or candy bar when trying to push through that mid-afternoon lull after a crappy night's sleep?

Lori laughed in understanding. "I've had to do everything in my power to resist afternoon cravings. Without the supplements you recommended for sugar cravings, I would have definitely given in and I'd probably be way heavier!"

Thankfully, Lori was on track with her eating, despite the increased cravings that her sleep deprivation was causing her. Sleep is connected to how we eat, what we eat, and how we feel. It's all connected: sleep, immunity, appetite, cravings, metabolism, weight...I think of it as a cycle because, oftentimes, better sleep leads to better eating and better eating leads to better sleep. Lori was eating her PFC-balanced meals and snacks throughout the day religiously, but she confessed that most of the time, she was skipping her bedtime snack. I would guess those were the nights she was sleeping the worst. I explained to her how skipping her bedtime snack would likely cause her to wake up in the middle of the night when her blood sugar levels go down. It all comes down to blood sugar stabilization. Blood sugars begin dropping after your last meal of the day, so to promote stable blood sugars all night long (which in turn promotes restful sleep), it's essential to bring your blood sugar levels back up slightly with a snack before bed. When you crash in the middle of the night, you have trouble sleeping.

Next, I checked in on her caffeine consumption. Her morning cup of coffee should be fine—problems arise when coffee is consumed all day long. Even a cup in the afternoon can interfere with sleep, and that's because the half-life of caffeine is around five or six hours. This means if you're relying on a cup of java to help you get through the afternoon, the caffeine could very well still be in your system at bedtime, interfering with your sleep. It's a vicious cycle that's all too common in the world today: coffee interfering with sleep and lack of sleep interfering with energy levels, thus causing you to consume more coffee, which interferes with your next night's sleep...It goes on and on. That's why it's helpful to figure out your individual "Coffee Cut-off" time—the time when you know that if you take in any amount of caffeine thereafter, it's likely to interfere with your sleep. (Mine's 2:00 pm.) The best way to figure this out is to track your sleep and when your last intake of caffeine was for the day before. Once you've determined your cut-off time, your best bet is to consume coffee before that time so you don't find yourself in the middle of this vicious cycle.

Another big sleep-saboteur is alcohol. In the last chapter we'll dive into exactly how alcohol can affect sleep. Lori wasn't a drinker, so this wasn't an issue for her.

The third factor I checked in on with Lori was what time she supplemented with Pure Magnesium. She said lately she'd been taking it in the afternoon to help kick chocolate cravings (glutamine helps fight sugar cravings, and magnesium is good for chocolate cravings specifically), and sometimes in the evening if she was feeling stiff after a long work day or workout, to relax her muscles. Magnesium is an important mineral—involved in over 300 different processes in the body (and essential for weight loss)—and most of us are deficient in it. Due to deterioration of soil minerals over the years, our food has less and less magnesium to offer. Magnesium deficiency can be the cause of sleep issues, chocolate cravings, muscle cramps, headaches, and more. Magnesium can be taken at a specific time in relation to what you are specifically using it for. Since it helps with sleep due to its calming and muscle-relaxing effects, allowing one to fall asleep faster and sleep more soundly, I recommended that she take an additional dose a half hour before bed, along with her bedtime snack.

Fortunately, Lori was totally onboard with that. She had come to realize the benefits of quality supplementation, though it wasn't always that way. When I first recommended supplementing with magnesium to help her with sore, stiff muscles and chocolate cravings, she had written me off and said she'd tried that before and it hadn't worked. I deduced that the problem was that she had taken a cheap magnesium supplement from the drugstore that was totally ineffective.

When she tried the VeroVive™ brand one, which I personally take myself and recommend to clients (with amazing results), she immediately started reaping the benefits.

Now, there are a number of other supplements that can help support sleep, too. Some people find magnesium does the trick, and others require additional support. You can get my guide with recommendations for sleep supplements, including the best brands, when to take them and how much to take, all at dietitiancassie.com/sleep.

My next tip for Lori to try was to minimize her blue light exposure. Researchers have known for a while that exposure to blue light—that light emitted by TV, computer, smartphone and tablet screens—around bedtime disrupts your body's melatonin production, which can interfere with sleep. Of course, a no-brainer solution to the late night technology dilemma would be to simply *turn it off*. Well, as you can imagine (and perhaps relate to), that's not always realistic. That's why I'm thankful to have found a handful of apps for electronic devices that have seriously saved my own sleep, the sleep of tons of our clients, and will likely save yours too!

The way they work is simple: they adjust the color of your screen to adapt to the time of day by filtering out blue light emitted by your device after sunset. You might be surprised because the change is so subtle, you don't necessarily even notice these apps gradually changing your screen's color. However, if you disable or pause it, you'll be shocked by how bright your screen gets! Personally, I didn't truly realize how much my evening technology use was interfering with my sleep until I set out to do something about it.

There are sleep apps for both iOS and Android devices that I love because they are both easy to use and really effective. I put the ones I recommend together for you in a guide, along with my other sleep tips, which you can also find at dietitiancassie.com/sleep.

If you get sleepy at the same time every night and wake up feeling like a million bucks every morning, consider yourself blessed because you are in the minority. Over half of all adults struggle with their sleep—the average American gets less than seven hours per night, when most of us need eight or nine. Sadly, inadequate sleep is all too common thanks to our busy, chaotic schedules. In fact, sometimes sleep may seem like a luxury. Lori's story is common. Too often, we see clients who seem to be eating all the right foods at the right times, but they're tossing and turning all night. Or, they're sleeping well, but only for five or six hours a night. Or they are sacrificing sleep for exercise—staying in the "calories in and calories out" mindset, which frankly *doesn't* help the weight situation. Giving up ZZZ's for exercise can interfere with your hormonal balance, which is critical for weight loss. I used to sacrifice sleep to hit the gym for hours on end, stuck in a hamster wheel of my own creation. Little did I know I was simply trading in one problem for another. It was a total waste and my suffering sleep schedule (along with too much exercise and not enough rest) likely caused inflammation, making my health spiral downwards while my weight went up. It's counterproductive to lose sleep in an attempt to spend more time on the treadmill, especially when simply snoozing more can help you lose weight. You can be doing everything else right, but if you're slacking on sleep, you're sabotaging your weight and health.

If you struggle with sleep, it's no wonder you're feeling tired, frustrated and having trouble with cravings, sickness and/or your weight. Sleep is the time for your body to build, regenerate, repair, and reset. Improving your sleep will improve your life. Whether you lay in bed for what seems like forever and can't seem to "turn off" your brain, or you fall asleep easily but then toss and turn in the middle of the night, or you wake up in the morning feeling unrested, the sleep recommendations I've outlined in my guide are for you. Go to dietitiancassie.com/sleep to download it for free. After some time and experimentation, they worked for Lori, and they can work for you too!

CHAPTER FOURTEEN

SUGAR: THE TRUTH ABOUT YOUR COOKIE, CAKE AND POTATO CHIP ADDICTION

"The worst part is that to lose the weight, I know what I need to do, I just can't seem to do it. It boils down to the fact that I don't have any willpower. I can't stop at just one." Wiping away the tracks of her tears, "I mean, my husband doesn't have this problem. He eats one piece of cake and he's done. Me, on the other hand? I can't stop until the whole darn thing is gone. Or until one of us chucks it into the garbage. And even then..." Her voice trailed off as she shook her head. We both knew why she didn't finish the sentence; it was too full of truth and shame.

"Jodi. Look at me," I said sternly. "It's important that you understand one thing: This is *not* your fault. It's *not* about willpower, at least not the way you think it is." She shifted her gaze toward me once again. "Seriously," I continued. "Your desire to eat sweet things is *not* a lack of willpower. It's not your fault that you have these cravings, and it's also not your fault that you give in. Let that soak in for a moment. I used to have those same thoughts, too. I know the feeling...all too well."

"It's taken over my life," Said Jodi. "I don't mean to be dramatic, but it's affecting my sleep—I toss and turn all night, and I know it's because of the bowl of ice cream before bed. It's affecting my work because I can't focus if I don't snack on junk food all day. Then, of course, when I do, it makes me feel defeated and worthless. I mean, I sometimes feel crazy...my relationships...my sex life..." She paused again and breathed deeply. After centering herself, she said, "It's like I'm not me! I feel powerless. I *literally* think about sugar of some kind or another all day long. The rare times I don't give into my cravings, I'm a monster, and when I do give in, I'm a disaster. I mean, I feel like a drug addict for something that is everywhere and seems to affect no one else but me. I think that I must just be weak. "

"Interesting that you mention drug addiction," I replied. "You may already know this, but sugar is like a drug. It has the same effect on the brain as cocaine. It triggers the same rewards centers. It's not only real, but for a lot of people— myself included, not so long ago—it's debilitating. Everything you're describing to me is a sugar addiction."

I thought about how much I could relate to Jodi. I can't count the number of times I tried to "get clean." Not from any drug—though it's affects on my body were just as damaging. I felt like a junkie. I would try to abstain, but then I needed my fix. "Just a quick hit. Then I'll feel better." But, just like Jodi, one hit—or bite—was never just one. Unlike those who are addicted to hard drugs, I was surrounded by my addiction. I could get it at any gas station, grocery store...heck, Amazon.com could send me some with same-day shipping! The drug is sugar. Any substance that had it sent my body into a chemical frenzy. I felt so out of control. I was a will-less Pavlovian dog. One whiff, or even just the thought of it, and I salivated.

I felt so alone at the time, as though I were the only one suffering, but now I know I wasn't. Perhaps you've felt this way, too? Thousands, maybe even millions, of us across the U.S. struggle with this, yet in our society, it's either laughed off (because sugar's pervasiveness has become commonplace and socially acceptable...even expected), or it's hidden behind closed doors because of the shame that accompanies it. Are you constantly thinking about where you'll get your next sugar fix, your next "guilty pleasure" or "cheat?" Are you trying to tune out that voice right now—the one telling you that you *need* another cookie, brownie, muffin, potato chip, or fill-in-the-blank-with-your-guilty-pleasure?

Did you catch that I mentioned potato chips there? That's because sugar cravings are not just about sweets. All carbohydrates turn into sugar in your body. You may not have a "sweet tooth," but when your blood sugar levels are low, if you grab potato chips or pretzels (or even just a slice or two of bread!) like they're going out of style, you're still a sugar addict. So, we're talking about obvious added sugars and also carbohydrates since they all turn into sugar in your body. The processed, refined carbohydrates turn into the most sugar. When you eat processed carbs like breads, pastas, cakes, crackers, granola bars, cereal, and potato chips, your blood sugar spikes high and fast, setting you up for a ride on the blood sugar roller coaster that causes inflammation and more cravings.

It's also important to be on the lookout for sneaky sugar lurking in foods that shouldn't have added sugar. There are way too many foods that fall into this category! Barbecue sauce, salad dressings, ketchup, chewing gum...several *vitamins* even have added sugar. Why? Because we're addicted, and food and supplement manufacturers and marketing companies alike know it and use it to their advantage. Without realizing it, the peanut butter you find yourself buying every week is one that has double the amount of sugar than the one you used to buy. We see this happening all the time with our clients and it's important to be on the defense. Our food system sets us up for failure when it comes to our weight and kicking sugar cravings.

You'll want to start reading labels to become aware of hidden sugars. Under the ingredient list, you're looking out for sugar, corn syrup, high fructose corn syrup (HFCS), evaporated cane juice, dehydrated cane syrup, fruit juice concentrate, barley malt, glucose solids, turbaned, maltodextrin, honey, molasses, maple syrup, and anything ending in -ose (fructose, sucrose, maltose, galactose, dextrose). That's a long list! What about honey, coconut sugar, agave nectar, or monk fruit sugar? Clients will ask this question because they are told that these are healthier, since they contain a few nutrients. My response is that sugar is sugar is sugar. It's all metabolized the same way in your body, whether it has more nutrients in it or not. (On that note, I don't think we should be getting our nutrients from sugar anyway!) It's all setting you up for that vicious cycle of cravings. So you may be not even be consciously feeding your addiction when dipping those chicken fingers in BBQ, but the truth is, there may be as much sugar in that BBQ sauce as there is in a Twinkie!

This was all a revelation to Jodi. "I know, calling your compulsion to consume sugar an addiction probably sounds a bit dramatic, but let me explain. Addiction is defined as the continued use of a mood-altering substance or behavior despite adverse dependency consequences. When you are addicted to something, you keep exposing yourself to it—

even when you know that it's harming your health. You said you can't stop after just one, right?"

"Right. That's exactly my problem," Jodi said.

"Exactly. When you respond to a sugar craving by having a cookie...or five...you find yourself experiencing a blood sugar spike followed by a crash well below a normal level. Your brain doesn't know what to make of these spikes and crashes, but it does know that low blood sugar levels are a problem. So, it sets off its emergency alarm system and tells you to eat more sugar! You dutifully do so, despite the feelings of shame. You eat another cookie...and then another, and another, setting you up on the addictive cycle. This results in repeated cycles of low blood sugar levels, increasing your tolerance for sugar, and programming your brain to want more and more and more. Being addicted to sugar is real, and the fact of the matter is that sugar cravings have *nothing* to do with a lack of willpower, and *everything* to do with balancing your brain chemistry."

At that point, Jodi interrupted saying that she just didn't think it was possible to cut sugar out of her life. The mere thought of it caused her anxiety. I acknowledged the fear she was feeling. After all, I'd been there. It was totally normal. Just like any addict would feel overwhelmed by the notion of going cold-turkey, a sugar addict is no different. There is good reason for it. We grow up with both physical *and* emotional attachments to this beast. It's common to feel some resistance to the idea of not having it as part of your daily routine...whether you're celebrating, or crying, or looking for a pick-me-up when you're exhausted. However, the sugar never really makes the celebration more meaningful. It never fixes the reason why you're crying. It never is a true pick-me up because it means you'll only be dropping to further depths in just a few short moments.

"Here's the truth," I told Jodi, "you can live a sugar-free life. I know it sounds crazy, but it is possible. Now, here's the even better news…You don't have to live sugar free! Unlike the heroin addict who can never have "just a little heroin," a sugar addict is able to abstain from sugar—clean out the body's system—and then, once the chemicals are balanced again, you will be able to enjoy the occasional indulgence, but this time without going off the deep end. Before we get you there, though, you must first understand how sugar behaves in the body and then, how you can manage it."

At this point, Jodi seemed to be coming around, but I knew I needed to give her a more tangible visual to fully appreciate the gravity of what was happening in her body.

The Shock of Sugar

"Think of sugar as little shards of glass that are cutting up your insides, thus inflaming your body, even if you can't feel it. It leads to weight gain and stops your weight loss in a couple of ways. First, when you consume sugar in excess, it's stored in your cells as fat, and second, when you have that sugar—those pieces of glass—inflaming your insides, it becomes a daily battle for your body until you give it a break. It focuses on putting this fire out before allowing you to lose weight. Besides, like you told me, your sugar consumption is affecting a lot more than just your waistline. For a lot of my other clients, it's been the culprit behind migraine headaches, feeling bloated, tossing and turning at night—like you said you are—and feeling mentally foggy all day. It's also caused relationship tension for some of my other clients, too."

"Of course," I told her, "I wouldn't expect you to 'just give it up.' I know you've tried that before and I had too, and we both know that doesn't work. That's exactly why it's not just about taking away your sugar. It's about addressing the underlying biochemical reasons for your sugar cravings."

"What do you mean by "biochemical reasons?" Jodi asked.

I always prefer to give people compelling visuals to help them understand the gravity of their nutritional decisions, so I again took the opportunity:

"Think of it this way. Let's say that your body is a building. You notice that there are cracks in the walls and ceilings. Each time you see a crack, you get plaster to mend it. However, the cracks keep showing up, so you keep plastering. Sooner or later, your walls and ceilings will be mostly just plaster. If you really want to fix the building, you'd look beyond the walls and examine the foundation. If the foundation is faulty, no amount of plaster will fix the cracks."

"Your biochemistry has had cracks in it. So, you've been plastering it with sugar. It never fixes the foundational problem of the base, imbalanced chemistry in your body. Now, the good news is that when a building has a faulty foundation, you might have to tear it down to rebuild. Thankfully, your body is a malleable organism that will learn to fix those root-cause chemical gaps with just a few adjustments of what you put into your body."

"Sugar cravings are a biochemical response in your brain. They are the response to one of two things—or both of them working together. These are the real reasons you get cravings in the first place. The first possible cause is low blood sugar levels. Your brain is really smart and knows that if your blood sugar levels are below where they should be, it wants to raise them—*stat*, and the quickest way it can bring them back up is if you consume sugar. As I'm sure you already know, it's virtually impossible to not give into sugar cravings when your brain is driving you to get your hands on sugar as fast as you possibly can. The other possible cause of your sugar cravings is that you don't have enough neurotransmitters, which is a fancy word for brain chemicals like dopamine, serotonin, and GABA. You need those to prevent those compelling sugar cravings from surfacing."

"Of course the exciting part about all of this is that there is something you can do about it. You don't have to live this way. Myself and thousands of our clients who have gone through my program have complete control over sugar cravings—even though we never thought it was possible."

Kick the Craving

"I'm finally shedding the pounds that I couldn't when I was giving into my sweet tooth!"

"I didn't know I could live life without craving sugar all day long every day."

"I never dreamed of a life without sugar cravings."

"I feel free for the first time in my life!"

These are direct quotes from an email from Jodi several months later, and they're exactly the kinds of things we hear from our clients every day as they are, for the first time in their lives, kicking their sugar cravings and reaping the benefits. So, let's take a look at how you can get there, too.

There are many steps to busting and preventing sugar cravings. I'll outline the first few so that you can get started right now, and you can download the rest, all of which I outlined in a free guide I created for you that can be found at dietitiancassie.com/bustsugarcravings.

The first thing you'll want to do, if you haven't implemented this just yet, is *get off that blood sugar roller coaster.* I outlined the best way to do this in the very first section of this book. "PFC Every Three" should be your motto. Eat a protein, fat, and carbohydrate every three to four hours. Focus on real, whole foods; the less packaged, processed and refined, the better. Snack between your meals, and have quality protein and healthy fat along with carbs every single time. This keeps sugar cravings at bay by keeping your blood sugar levels nice and stable, so that you don't hit those lows where your brain tells you to fix it by eating sugar. Remember, when you don't eat for long periods of time, your blood sugar levels crash, and that's one of the reasons why you crave sugar.

Breaking this step down even further, the simplest way to do this is to intentionally eat more healthy fat and protein. This alone will make it easier to eat fewer carbohydrates and less sugar. For me, and for so many of our clients who come in craving sugar like no other, this simple step works wonders immediately. Healthy fat and protein keep your blood sugar levels balanced so you stay satisfied and full and your desire for sugar diminishes. When you do this, a hormonal message (cholecystokinin) is sent to your brain to tell you to stop eating. Fat specifically slows down the absorption of sugar into your bloodstream so that you don't get a huge surge that is followed by a *crash* which is when you crave sugar. Protein helps in an extra special way because it is a precursor for your neurotransmitters—the brain chemicals I mentioned earlier— that you need adequate amounts of to keep sugar cravings at bay. You can support the production of these neurotransmitters by consuming protein throughout the day— not just at meal time but an ounce or two for snacks as well. Shoot for a couple tablespoons of healthy fats like butter, avocado, olives, nuts and seeds, along with a few ounces of meat, fish or a couple of eggs for protein.

While your food choices are absolutely important for managing your cravings, there's more to it than that. As I mentioned earlier, I don't expect you to be able to "just stop eating sugar" without first addressing your underlying biochemical imbalance. That's where key supplementation comes into play. Supplementation is a critical and often overlooked part of the battle with sugar cravings. We can certainly balance our blood sugar levels with food, but our clients struggling with frequent, intense sugar cravings find that food alone isn't enough to keep the cravings away for good. This is where balancing your biochemistry comes into play. If you try to break free of your cravings with nutrients from food alone, you may have some success, but ultimately when you are sugar sensitive, your body won't be completely craving-free if you aren't supporting it with the nutrients it is lacking on a long-term basis. This is something I learned the hard way until I finally realized I couldn't control my cravings with just food, so I make it a priority to start supporting my brain and body by supplementing every single day. Supplementing is a critical part of battling the sugar dragon and may be, in fact, the most powerful, life-changing step for you and for your weight loss. The guide I referenced above outlines the key supplements for preventing sugar cravings, and you can download it for free at dietitiancassie.com/bustsugarcravings.

In addition to supplementing, stress management helps to keep sugar cravings away, too. The connection between stress and sugar cravings is powerful for a few key reasons. First, cortisol (your "stress hormone") is released in response to stress. It raises your blood sugar levels, and when they crash, that is when you crave. Also, stress can weaken your gut lining, making it more permeable and thus interfering with production of those important neurotransmitters (brain chemicals) that you need to have enough of so that you don't crave sugar.

The last thing you absolutely *must* know about beating sugar cravings and getting on the road to weight loss is that it's a strength to ask for support. While overcoming the sugar cravings is absolutely liberating and rewarding, it's likely going to prove extremely challenging, too. If you have been running on a sugar high for a long time, the breakthrough process can be like overcoming a drug addiction which can include frustration, withdrawals, and even relapses. This is all normal. Don't look past getting support from a licensed healthcare professional with experience in overcoming sugar addiction. You can have all the right tools, but a lot of times we find that it's the individualized guidance and accountability that pushes our clients through to the other side. My team and I are here for you to help support and guide you through this process. You can get in touch with us at healthysimplelife.com.

Again, for my full list of tools and a beautiful printable guide that we use with our clients to conquer cravings, check out dietitiancassie.com/bustsugarcravings.

CHAPTER FIFTEEN

SWEETENERS: YAY OR NAY?

Now that we've beaten sugar into the ground, we can't go on without discussing a related key to unlocking stubborn weight loss…something that could be the very thing you've replaced sugar with in an honest attempt to be healthier and lose weight. Similar to supplements as we discussed earlier, many people are ingesting these in an attempt to do their body good because they think it will help with weight loss. In reality, they're doing the opposite and not only hindering weight loss, but causing weight *gain*, among other problems. They're found in all sorts of things from protein bars to chewing gum, cough drops, soda, and even *vitamins*.

Yes, the nasty culprits I'm talking about are artificial sweeteners, which also go by another undercover name: sugar substitutes. All of them—saccharin, sucralose (commonly known as Splenda), aspartame—they're all artificial, and they all have some serious consequences associated with their consumption, including weight gain, which is ironic since their main marketing claim is weight loss. Let's take a step back and ask ourselves, might there be a connection between the sugar substitute craze and the rising obesity rates? Doesn't it seem too good to be true that foods could taste so sweet and have no negative effect on the body? If it does, that's because it is.

Here's why artificial sweeteners backfire: The original logic and promise behind using artificial sweeteners in place of sugar is that they contain no calories, so they'll help you shed pounds. With this "magnificent" discovery, these magical substances were added to various foods in place of sugar and/or fat to reduce the caloric value. You can find them in products like diet soda, light yogurt, powdered drink mixes, canned fruit, low-fat ice cream, chewing gum, and as I mentioned, even vitamins. They are usually in products that flaunt eye-catching terms like: *sugar-free, light, lower calorie, diet, reduced sugar, zero,* or the one I dislike most: *skinny.* This promise to fulfill your fantasy of getting all the sweet while the pounds melt away is an empty one. We know already that weight loss is not just a matter of calories in and calories out.

Here's the hidden problem. *Because* artificial sweeteners contain no calories, they mess up your metabolism. That's right, these phony substances actually confuse your metabolism which in turn slows it down and leads to weight gain—exactly the opposite effect you're wanting when attempting to forgo the calories you get from real sugar.

To make matters worse, not only do artificial sweeteners *not* help you lose weight, but they're also quite dangerous. Artificial sweetener consumption is continually associated with metabolic syndrome—a term used to refer to a group of risk factors that occur together and increase the risk for heart disease, stroke, and type 2 diabetes—not good. When the

American Diabetes Association is publishing and standing behind these facts (Nettleton, 2009)[4], we know we should be extra concerned! Artificial sweeteners also negatively impact our gut health by killing off the good bacteria, which, as we discussed in part two of this book, is needed for health and weight loss. When that good bacteria is wiped out, it damages your gut and leaves it inflamed—the last thing you want if you're trying to lose weight. Virtually all of us should be working on healing our guts, especially when the desired result is weight loss. So, the last thing we want to do is consume something that's further impairing our gut health (which is exactly what using artificial sweeteners do).

As we discussed in the last chapter, we are learning more and more about the addictive nature of sugar. This could be the case with artificial sweeteners, too. Studies have suggested they increase our appetite and desire for sweetness since they can trigger the same reward center in the brain that sugar does…except your body never actually gets the sugar, so it's never satisfied. So, using artificial sweeteners as a replacement for sugar might make us eat more sugar *anyway*. These artificial sweeteners aren't helping you battle those cravings; they're exacerbating them!

Plus, they're gross. Splenda contains chlorine. *Three* chlorine molecules to be exact. I can hardly stand swimming in a pool with chlorine for very long because that smell makes me gag, not to mention how it makes my eyes burn. I certainly don't want to be ingesting it!

Now, if you've been using them, don't feel guilty. I used to abuse them too, thinking they were the lesser of two evils when compared to sugar. Before I un-brainwashed myself from the artificial sweetener fallacy I learned in dietitian

---

[4] Nettleton, JA. "Diet Soda Intake and Risk of Incident Metabolic Syndrome ..." 2009. <http://care.diabetesjournals.org/content/32/4/688.full>

school, I would scratch my head in wonder why a client wouldn't lose a single pound after they replaced a 12-pack of soda with a 12-pack of diet (artificially sweetened) soda. Even more confusing—more often than not, in fact—the said client would gain weight. I always found it peculiar that thousands of calories could just be magically slashed, yet a person still wouldn't lose weight. But that's just it: at the time, we thought calories were all there was to look at. Now we know that weight isn't just dictated by calories, and we *also* know that ingesting chemicals made in a lab can cause weight gain. Artificial sweeteners are *far* from being healthy and guilt-free like they've been touted by manufacturing companies, marketing schemes, and even dietitians.

So, throw away your pink, yellow and blue packets!

So what is the solution? In place of these, I suggest using either plain ol' sugar or pure stevia. Stevia is a natural sweetener that comes from a plant rather than a lab—and it's 30 times sweeter than sugar, so you don't have to use much. Just be sure it's not Truvia—the gold standard of well-executed false advertising. We've been led to believe that Truvia is the same thing as Stevia, and the (disappointing) truth is that, despite the fact that Truvia is marketed as a "stevia-based sugar substitute," it is not the same thing. Not even close, actually. The ingredient list for Truvia is as follows: Erythritol, Rebiana, and Natural Flavors. Just three ingredients, and stevia isn't even one of them! Truvia is mostly erythritol, a sugar alcohol. On that note, I am not a fan of sugar alcohols in general. (Xylitol, Erythritol, Maltitol, Sorbitol—they usually end in "ol"). Our bodies do a poor job of digesting sugar alcohols, and because they aren't completely digested, they hang out in our intestines where they are fermented by colonic bacteria. They are notorious for their unpleasant side effects, so for a lot of people, this leads to gastric distress, diarrhea, cramping, gas, and bloating.

Those side effects can lead to inflammation, which we've talked enough about already, and for that reason, I recommend avoiding them.

Back to stevia! For the record, I still wouldn't consider stevia a free pass to the all-you-can-consume buffet, since it could still increase your desire for sweetness. That said, it has been around long enough for us to know that it's a safe alternative to sugar.

In summary, artificial sweeteners don't deliver on any of their intended promises. They contribute to weight gain, even if they're calorie free. They worsen gut health. They can even make us eat more sugar. *What's the point?* Why play tricks on your body when they end up backfiring anyway? Because we have been brainwashed by marketing campaigns for so many years, it's important to change our mindsets about how we think about sugar and nutrition. Start by remembering that your body was designed to metabolize food, not chemicals. It is better to eat a little bit of the real thing (sugar) than a lot of the fake thing (chemicals). Think of eating as a way to give your body energy, because that's exactly what you are doing every time you eat. Choose to steer clear of the sweeteners and fuel with foods that are high in nutrients and low in additives and chemicals. Keep it simple. Focus on real, whole foods and don't buy into marketing tactics for artificially sweetened things.

If you feel like you "need" something sweeter, check in with yourself: Why do we "need" these sweeteners anyway? Could it be because we are excessively addicted to sugar? Do your best to keep the focus on real food, and if you find that to be nearly impossible due to your sugar cravings, be sure to also implement my tips to break the sugar addiction from the last chapter and as outlined in my free guide at dietitiancassie.com/bustsugarcravings.

PART 4

AMPLIFY YOUR EFFORTS

CHAPTER SIXTEEN

THE BEST PART OF THE DAY

Are you skipping the best part of the day?

When I was a kid, as much as I despised bedtime like most kids do, there was something bittersweet about it. Bedtime was directly preceded by my absolute most favorite part of the day: The Bedtime Snack!

From the moment I started eating dinner, the wheels in my brain would begin turning as I would think about what I wanted for that special, scrumptious snack. My last chance to eat. The BEST part of the day. I had to make it count. I'd be plopped in front of the TV watching a cartoon, and I knew by the third commercial break, I would hear the sweet announcement from my mom that it was time for my final treat of the day. Those words were like magic to my ears, and I would jump up from my seat and bolt to the cupboard, drooling with excitement as I carefully selected what I would devour.

Back then I had ice cream, cookies, crackers, cereal, or popcorn...all the typical bedtime snacks. Of course, these are all the same snacks that leave us with gut rot and bog down our metabolism. None of them are ideal, but *especially* not before bed—it's the last thing your body should have before you lie flat on your back for seven or, ideally, eight hours (even more for kids). The wrong bedtime snack will slow down your metabolism. Did you know that the *right* one can speed it up? Oh yes. You heard me right. This is why I'm telling you to bring back The Bedtime Snack!

We've been misled for far too long that a bedtime snack is a sin. You may have been told over and over again that eating before bed will make you fat, that eating before bed provides unnecessary calories, and you shouldn't eat after some specific time. This is widespread, well-known, *and* a total myth. It's true that satisfying your sweet tooth with a sugary snack can pack on the pounds, but not all snacks are created equal. In fact, a bedtime snack will actually support you in reaching your weight loss goal, so long as it's the *right* type of snack.

The bedtime snack has been a weight loss lifesaver for countless clients of ours. While I knew it was important, I didn't truly see the effectiveness until Carol came along. Carol was a client of mine for eight months before she embraced the bedtime snack. She was following all of my recommendations to a T...except for this one. I don't know if I brushed over the importance of it too quickly, or if it didn't register with her how crucial it was, or maybe she didn't admit that she just wasn't doing it, but the fact of the matter remained: the bedtime snack was not part of her routine. We were eight months into her plan, and she was still pounds away from her weight loss goal. I was determined to get to the bottom of it, so I took out my magnifying glass. At that point, we had covered all of the key practices for losing weight that I typically focus on with my clients (and have laid out in detail in the chapters of this book for you) for several months. As we were walking through her typical day, everything seemed right—until I asked her what happened after dinner. She looked at me with a blank stare through that computer webcam and said matter-of-factly, "Nothing. That's when I read my book, have a cup of tea, and eventually go to bed."

I said, "What about the bedtime snack?" That's when the lightbulb turned on for me. For Carol, though, it wasn't that fast.

Through my computer screen, I could see she her shrug her shoulders and say, "I guess I'm never really hungry after dinner. My cup of tea seems to hold me over just fine." This is when things started to get fun. But first, I had to get Carol onboard.

How the Bedtime Snack Works

She didn't quite understand how the bedtime snack actually promotes weight loss. In the back of her mind, she was still considering the bedtime snack to be "unnecessary calories." We know that's not how it works, though. It all comes down to blood sugar stabilization. Blood sugars begin dropping after your last meal of the day, so to promote stable blood sugars all night long and ensure you are a fat-burning machine while you sleep, it's essential to bring your blood sugar levels back up slightly with a snack before bed.

The ideal bedtime snack includes healthy fat and nutrient-dense carbohydrates (i.e. veggies and fruits). Note that the bedtime snack is the only time I recommend only two parts of my PFC mantra. I don't recommend protein as it can boost your metabolism so much that it can keep you from falling asleep. So skip the P! What I've found to work best for most people is fifteen minutes to half an hour before bed, have a small bowl of frozen berries (half a cup or so) topped with two or three tablespoons of heavy cream.

Here are a few other bedtime snack ideas:

- A cup or two of raw carrots and a half or quarter cup of guacamole.

- Half of a sliced apple with a couple tablespoons of almond or cashew butter.

- Half of a sweet potato with a couple tablespoons of butter or coconut oil, topped with cinnamon.

- Half of a pear sautéed in coconut oil and topped with coconut milk and walnuts.

Now, try to stick with a couple tablespoons (or half an avocado) of fat, and a half cup (or half of a sweet potato or half of an apple) of carbs. If you're tired or lazy, a handful of nuts and a handful of dried fruit will do the trick, too!

The bedtime snack means you don't have to push through that hungry feeling and go to bed on an empty stomach! And, even if you're not hungry, it's still important to eat a snack to reap the metabolism boosting and weight-loss benefits!

I emphasized to Carol the importance of having a bedtime snack, even if she wasn't hungry. It's not about halting hunger as much as it is about bringing your blood sugar levels back up so they're nice and stable all night long. Even if it was a handful of sunflower seeds and a handful of blueberries with that cup of tea, it had to happen in order for her metabolism to stay active. She went along with it, but didn't seem too convinced.

Two weeks later, I called her for her next appointment and she exclaimed, "I can't believe it! I'm losing weight again!" This continued for months until she reached her weight loss goal.

Throughout the process, Carol asked me to give her the recap on the bedtime snack a couple more times. She said she was trying to explain to her husband how she could change one simple thing and lose more weight, especially when this one simple thing is something that goes against what we've been taught for so many years. She also pointed out that with the addition of this snack, she's eating more food in general. It was the missing link—she needed to add more fuel to keep her metabolism running—just what she needed to shed those extra pounds.

Nowadays, I still look forward to my bedtime snack just like I did as a child, but it's not just because I like it. It promotes restful sleep, keeps my metabolism in high gear, and helps me to start out the next day on the right foot—and it can do the same for you! Consuming a bedtime snack is not only the best way to end your day, but it also sets you up for success for the next day, too!

A lot of our clients find that the nights they toss and turn are the same ones they forgot to have a bedtime snack, or had an unbalanced one that spiked their blood sugar levels, causing them to crash in the middle of the night. No wonder a lot of us have sleep issues. Imagine trying to sleep on a roller coaster! Impossible, right? That's what happens when you have a bedtime snack that spikes your blood sugar levels right before you go to sleep. As you learned in an earlier chapter, sleep quality is one of the hidden keys to unlocking that stubborn weight loss. Sometimes it takes finding one key in order to discover the next.

CHAPTER SEVENTEEN

EXERCISE:
DON'T WASTE YOUR TIME

"I just don't get it. I do my best to eat well and bust my tail at the gym six or even seven days a week, which is more than any of my friends or coworkers. I burn so many calories, and yet not only have I not *lost* any weight, but I've actually *gained* a pound. It doesn't make sense, and it's embarrassing. I hate it!"

I didn't know much about Katie yet, this was her first appointment with me, but I completely understood her frustration. To be investing all the time, energy, and effort, only to end up heavier than when she started...What gives!?

Maybe you can relate. Maybe you too are diligently slaving away at the gym, day in and day out, and you still haven't lost a pound. Worse yet, maybe you're like Katie and you're actually gaining weight in spite of your best efforts.

I nodded my head in understanding and reassured her, "You're certainly not the first client to walk through those doors with the same frustrations and the same predicament. What's happening in your body is something you don't hear about from weight loss experts or the media. In fact, they're telling us the opposite; the calorie-counting myth continues to spread even though, as you're experiencing, weight loss simply doesn't work that way."

I told Katie that in the journey of weight loss, nutrition is of far greater importance than fitness. Abs really are made in the kitchen—it's a saying that has stuck around for good reason. There was a time not so long ago when you could have told me this and I wouldn't have believed you. At the same time, as a former marathon runner, I always did find it peculiar that people could train for and run marathons—which meant thousands and thousands of calories burned over the course of weeks and months of training—yet they wouldn't shed a pound. In fact, just like with Katie, sometimes the opposite would happen.

The Cardio Conundrum

During my marathon running days, I led a running group. This meant hours and hours of conversations with fellow marathon trainees, many of whom were on a quest for weight loss, which is what compelled them to start running in the first place. Several of my fellow runners would express their frustration when they ended up heavier after the marathon than before they started training. How is it possible to gain weight during the training and completion of a marathon? Sometimes they would have the hopeful thought, "Well, maybe I just gained muscle. Since muscle weighs more than fat, that's where the pounds came from." That was rarely—if ever—the case. Then you'd think the number on the scale would be lower after burning all those calories. Unfortunately, that's just not how it works. You've been told the key to weight loss is burning more than you're consuming in order to create a calorie deficit, but if that were the truth, then how come so many people are in Katie's shoes?

Burn more calories than you take in and you'll lose weight. In the same way, we've also been told the opposite: Consume more calories than you're burning and you'll gain weight. With that in mind, it's no wonder we spend hours upon hours running or "ellipticaling" to burn as many calories as we can. Nowadays, more people have gym memberships than ever before, yet we're also fatter than we've ever been. To this day, there hasn't been a single study showing that exercise alone causes significant weight loss (and certainly not sustainable weight loss). There's so much more to it than that.

One of the main reasons that burning tons of calories through exercise can still result in not losing a pound is because of a couple things we discussed earlier: cortisol and inflammation. Too much exercise is a stressor, and stress causes your body to release that stress hormone, cortisol. Cortisol spikes your blood sugar levels and that sugar gets stored as fat. That's part of it. The other part is the inflammation you create in your body from too much exercise. Too much exercise could actually be what's blocking your weight loss because of these reasons. As we discussed earlier, a little inflammation here and there is okay, and even normal, as your body is good at taking care of it. After exercising on a daily basis, you've got to understand there is an abundance of inflammation happening that your body isn't getting a break from. This would explain not only your inability to lose weight—as you're body is constantly fighting fires inside of you—but it's also why you're gaining weight, with all the compounding inflammation and sugar being stored as fat as a result of cortisol being triggered. Rest and recovery are crucial after tough workouts, and after a long pattern of exercising without sufficient recovery. Katie's body needed a period of time dedicated to just this.

I explained all of this to Katie and told her, "Katie, in order for you to lose weight, it's going to be critical for you to take a break from the marathons and allow your body a chance to rest and heal."

She sighed, exasperated. "It's crazy. Here I've been doing what I thought were all the right things to lose weight, and now you're telling me that it's all just been pushing my goals further out of reach? Why is everything so hard!?"

All I could do was nod my head in solidarity and understanding because it really is a frustrating and confusing topic. As you may have experienced yourself, or at the very least are seeing now as you're working through the chapters of this book, many of the things we've been told about weight loss aren't helpful, and they can flat out backfire. I know too many people who follow restrictive diets, counting calories or grams of fat, depriving their body of what it needs, all while putting it through hell at the gym—sometimes twice a day. Maybe you're one of them.

I can relate. I came to a point where I had to make a personal choice to change the type of exercise I participated in. I used to wake up at 4:00 in the morning to get to the gym and run for an hour on the treadmill before I instructed a 6:00 am bootcamp workout where I worked up a sweat for another hour. I did that almost every day for years. My body wasn't in any better shape back then, and it certainly wasn't as healthy. Despite my hard efforts, it was continually inflamed and bloated. I exercised more and gained more weight at the same time. I was in school for dietetics and exercise science and diligently doing what was considered "healthy." What was happening?

This inflammatory exercise regimen I was putting myself through continued as I started running marathons in an attempt to shed some of the pounds I was gaining. Besides, running a marathon was on my bucket list. I planned on the "one and done" strategy, but because I'm competitive, one marathon turned into four, and soon there came a point when I had to again step back and reassess what's healthy and what's not. Something didn't feel right. Was what I was putting my body through even "working?"

However, before I gave it up, I too had to be convinced that it wasn't healthy. At the time, my head was buried in research. When I came across the studies on this topic, I honestly didn't want to believe what I was finding, but there it was: Long durations of cardiovascular activity on a regular basis can cause inflammation, which is at the root of most diseases. I went on to explore how that tied into weight loss and weight gain. Essentially, inflammation drains your metabolism's energy because your body is focused on healing it. "Chronic cardio," as it was referred to, can also increase your body's production of cortisol—your stress hormone—setting you up for weight gain by raising blood sugar levels and triggering the release of insulin, your fat-storing hormone. At that point, I finally understood that you can gain weight from the stress you're putting on your body from doing something you've always been told would *help* with weight loss. What!?

"But isn't running supposed to be healthy?" I kept repeating to myself. Besides, I had come to enjoy running—it was a good outlet for me—a stress reliever. It gave me something to strive for and made me feel accomplished. And I worked up a sweat while doing it. It all seemed perfect. The problem though, based on what I was reading, was that running can actually cause stress in your body, hurting more than helping. The same is true for any type of exercise that you do at a lower intensity for a long time. All of those people you see at the gym on the elliptical machine for upwards of an hour are giving themselves gold stars when they are actually doing more harm than good. When you do this every single day, you're just making your body fight and fight and fight. That isn't good. If you are putting in long hours of endurance activity every day and don't give yourself a break, how do you expect your body to recover? Your body is good at healing itself, but do you really want it to spend all of its resources on healing instead of giving you energy that leads to weight loss, not to mention a higher quality of life? Every time your body is inflamed, it focuses on healing that inflammation as its top priority. Not weight loss. Not energy. Not happiness. Just healing.

I took a deep breath and sat with my thoughts, examining them with an honest heart. This made sense. It explained why there are overweight marathon runners and it explains why so many people can work so hard at the gym and not lose a pound, despite their best efforts.

As I kept reading and researching, I found that the best exercise for your metabolism, energy and weight loss is simple. High bursts of intense exercise for a little while— which I'll explain shortly—with adequate rest in-between. Then, give your body breaks and time to heal between each workout. When you push yourself with workouts five or more days a week, your body can adapt, but the lack of time to heal your muscles backfires with inflammation. Everyone's threshold is different of course, but the concept is the same: listen to your body and let it recover. Also, stop doing low-intensity exercise for a long time. It's not only ineffective for your weight loss and energy levels, but sadly it's also just a waste of time. It's not helping the number on the scale and the inflammation it promotes is at the root of diseases like heart disease, so it's not healthier for your heart or and it's not contributing to disease prevention at all.

Now, just like it's downright mean to restrict your body of the nutrients it needs (like fat or calories), subjecting your body to a constant state of inflammation is dishonoring, too. I want to treat my body with respect on a daily basis so that it rewards me by working to the best of its ability—giving me energy, crystal-clear focus, positive moods and glowing skin, hair and nails. That means I need to give my body periods of rest and recovery, and listen to it rather than doing things to it that it doesn't like. So, I reevaluated what this balance and honoring my body could look like for me. It could look slightly different for you—I'm not saying you can't exercise daily or wake up at 4am to go to the gym—but maybe there is something you can learn and apply from my experience.

Once I changed my exercise regimen, I started losing weight. Twenty pounds came off effortlessly with the change in my exercise regimen along with the addition of quality vitamin supplements that I hadn't been taking up to that point. Fast forward to now: I eat more calories and fat than ever before, I'm exercising far less than I have at any point in my life thus far, and I'm in the best shape of my life. I don't tell you that to brag, but because I used to believe getting in shape was 50% exercise + 50% nutrition, and now I know nutrition matters much more—and that "equation" is so much more heavily weighted in favor of proper nutrition than we ever thought (more like 80% nutrition, 20% exercise!). I still exercise, just not as much, and the exercise I do looks a lot different than it used to.

Exercise for Real Results

Back to Katie: I told her that giving up her daily gym time didn't mean she had to completely stop exercising. What it did mean was cutting back a lot in order to allow her body to heal, and then she could gradually add in different types of workouts.

"So what types of exercise can I do?" she immediately wanted to know.

I was glad she asked, because it meant she was still thinking about her physical wellness. Exercise isn't a bad thing in and of itself. In fact, while I don't promote exercise for the purpose of calorie burning, certain ones can be the hidden key that pushes you through your weight loss plateau. The right types of exercise can be incredibly beneficial for boosting metabolism, so the takeaway here is that not all types of exercise are created equal. It's the chronic, repetitive, daily endurance activity that is counterproductive and inflammatory.

I answered Katie's question like this: "First, I think you should step away from intense workouts for a couple weeks, and embrace yoga, pilates, and lower intensity exercises. While these are not the kinds that directly boost your metabolism, they will get you on track with your weight loss goal by giving your body time to heal before you crank it up again."

She seemed receptive, so I continued, "After a couple weeks of this, I recommend adding in short bursts of activity at high intensity intervals, a few times a week, to support your metabolism. High intensity interval workouts are alternating short periods of intense exercise with recovery periods. It's as simple as doing some exercise and then resting. These high intensity interval training workouts are the kind that really turbocharge your metabolism, and as a bonus: they don't require great lengths of time...also awesome." At that, she smiled. In our busy day and age, everyone loves when you give them some time back in their routine.

For your intervals, you can mix it up by including sets of both cardiovascular activity and resistance (strength) training to keep your heart pumping and your muscles strong, too. Jumping jacks, mountain climbers and running up and down the stairs count for cardio, and squats, pushups and lunges are more strength training exercises. Burpees and squat jumps are both! What I personally do and recommend you work up to is to set your stopwatch for 30 seconds. Do sets of these and any other moves you love with 30 seconds on and then a 30-second break in between sets. The break is to allow your body to rest so that you can push yourself hard again, but not so long that it fully recovered between sets. You can do 20 seconds on and 40 seconds off, or 15 seconds on and a 45-second break, especially when you first start this regimen, or when you're beginning to feel tired, like toward the end of your workout. You can start with just a few minutes of this and work your way up to 10 or 15 minutes at a time, based on how your body feels.

Considering Katie's goal of weight loss, this is what I told her to do: start with three to five minutes of this interval workout a few days a week, with the goal of doing ten or fifteen minutes, three times a week. This type of workout can be done at home without going to a gym, and when the weather is nice, you can do the same type of thing outside—30-second intervals, alternating between running and walking. You can find workouts structured around interval training at gyms and fitness centers, too. Usually they're called Tabata or HIIT— read the class descriptions and look for interval training!

I told Katie that intensity is more important than frequency. This may be the simplest metabolism-boosting switch that you can make: changing from the long, slow, boring, hamster-wheel workouts to shorter bursts of high intensity intervals with rest days in-between to properly recover! This type of exercise gives your metabolism a jump-start without causing stress in the body—exactly what Katie needed.

All exercise can produce an inflammatory response and a slowed metabolism if you're doing too much, so make your workouts harder (not longer), and not more frequent. Make sure you are well rested so that you can do harder workouts, albeit shorter ones. Exercising in this way supports your metabolism the most without promoting inflammation.

The optimal amount and frequency of exercise is different for everyone, but you can bet that if you're doing too much of it and not giving your body a chance to rest, the physical stress you're putting on yourself won't be doing you any metabolism-boosting favors, and it'll interfere with your weight loss goal. Above all, remember to always listen to your body, and when in doubt, less is more!

"What about cardio kickboxing classes?" she asked. That was a great question, especially because I know that for a lot of people, these classes are popular. I told her that it really depends on the structure of the class. If it's aligned with the interval principle, even a few minutes working hard and then breaking in-between, I think that's great! The problem is that a lot of workout classes are based on the long duration, low to mid intensity for the entire length of the class, which is the same problem as marathon running. While I don't see the harm in attending a class like this on occasion, I think it can be a problem when it becomes a regular occurrence. I told Katie, just like I had advised her to take a break from "chronic cardio", that I'd also suggest skipping any workouts that are done for long periods of time.

"You know what I like about this? I may actually enjoy having some free time again!" she said with a smile.

I nodded in agreement. "I totally understand!" While I'm all for making sacrifices and devoting oneself to something, I don't want anything to take over my life. I see that happen with a lot of people when they get obsessive about exercising for the sole purpose of burning calories…which doesn't work anyway. I was excited that Katie could already see another positive side of spending less time at the gym. Exercise can be an all-consuming endeavor, and finding the right balance is key to not only metabolism and weight loss, but also quality of life, too. You don't need to hit the gym daily to be healthy or fit, and you may even enjoy life more without being so strict about that.

As you shift away from long workouts, it's a wise idea to invest that extra time into planning and prepping your meals and snacks to bring you closer to your weight goals. In fact, at an initial client appointment, it isn't rare for us to ask them to spend less time at the gym and more time in their kitchen, making healthy food a priority, instead of trying to "burn off" junky stuff they eat when they're in a hurry.

I recommend focusing on food first. That's why this is one of the last chapters of the book. Exercise is still important, but it's not your first priority when weight loss is your goal. You can be torching calories left and right doing grueling workouts at the gym, but consuming excessive amounts of processed carbohydrates ultimately inhibits your ability to access and burn stored body fat. You can't just "burn off" the inflammatory foods you're eating. It doesn't work that way. You will not lose weight through exercising unless you are also moderating insulin production and taking care of the food part. Remember, insulin is your fat-storing hormone. Your pancreas will release it and it will do its job of storing fat— which it's really good at—whenever you eat processed carbs and sugar. You can exercise all day and all night long (as some of us have done, and may still be doing), but until you reduce your body's need for and release of insulin, you won't be losing weight. The first step to controlling this is ingesting less sugar, and the easiest way to make this happen is to eat more healthy fat and protein (read: PFC balance!). Invest time into balancing your eating and embrace a naturally active lifestyle—taking the stairs, parking in the furthest spot, walking the dog regularly, all while incorporating short bursts of brief, intense exercise.

This is what I encouraged Katie to do. To spend more time in the kitchen and to also do more physical activity of any kind that she enjoys—both during her couple weeks of rest and after that as part of her lifestyle. Moving more as part of your lifestyle will benefit you more than hours at the gym. Weed the garden, go for a bike ride, walk the dog, play tennis, practice handstands! For me, it's paddle boarding, yoga, rock-climbing, hiking, skiing, rollerblading, and biking. I also incorporate a few short interval training workouts during the week to mix it up. I still run on occasion, but my runs fall into the two to four mile length that makes me feel awesome afterward. Otherwise, I just do the interval workout style I outlined before. I've also created a makeshift standing desk for my work space to help negate some of the harmful effects of sitting all day long. There are several types of standing desks available, or you can create your own with a big stack of books! Overall, the goal is to move and to lead an active lifestyle...as best as you can in this sedentary world. The more you move, the better you'll feel and it is a good idea to mix the interval training in with your daily activity when your goal is weight loss.

So, you're probably wondering: what happened to Katie after she followed my recommendations? Well, I'm happy to report that she lost 25 pounds(!) in the following four months after incorporating interval workouts a few times a week instead of killing herself with longer, low-intensity cardio sessions. She is feeling great, and loves her new workout schedule! It's fun, energizing and she feels healthy and says she feels more balanced because she has more free time these days to do other things that she loves, too. Maybe you could benefit from implementing some of the things Katie found to help her. Maybe exercising smarter, not harder, is the key to unlocking that stubborn weight loss for you.

You might also be wondering about nutrition for exercise and the vitamins I alluded to earlier. I've created a guide to fueling and supplementing your workout and recovery, which is available for you to check out at dietitiancassie.com/exercise.

CHAPTER EIGHTEEN

CHEERS TO YOUR WEIGHT LOSS: WHEN AND WHEN NOT TO HIT HAPPY HOUR

Lisa is a career woman with two small children at home. When she rushed into my office, five minutes late and out of breath, one of the first things to come out of her mouth was, "Every day, I run around like a chicken with my head cut off—frantic, scatter-brained, and exhausted. I want you to know that I'll do everything in my power to eat whatever you want me to, but I won't give up my red wine. I'm no alcoholic, but I look forward to at least one glass when I get home. I deserve it with how hard I work and what I have to put up with all day long between work, my husband, and my kids!"

Lisa was here to lose weight. She was a yo-yo dieter. Every week, she was putting in way more hours at the office than her peers to get ahead. She was taking on more and more responsibilities and obligations in her many roles, and somehow she was just barely managing to accomplish all of this without neglecting her primary focus: her family. Of course, she did all this at the expense of her own health, barely having the time to focus on one nutritional plan before life got chaotic again and her attempts proved fruitless.

While she certainly didn't have an incredible amount of weight to lose, the pounds she wanted to shed were stubborn ones. Even the "best" diet on the planet would only cause her to lose them and gain them right back once life became too chaotic to keep up with it. Life was chaotic most of the time for Lisa. She was waking up every morning feeling exhausted, even if she clocked eight or even nine hours in her bed.

After analyzing Lisa's situation, I had to break the news to her that the best thing she could do for her waistline would be to get rid of alcohol altogether. Your body sees alcohol as a toxin, so when you drink it, your liver's primary goal is to detoxify and get rid of it. When your liver is focusing on metabolizing alcohol, it puts fat burning on the back burner. It also makes it harder to manage blood sugar levels— something Lisa had been working so hard at! Alcohol also promotes inflammation and interferes with your ability to sleep.

Lisa looked at me with a furrowed brow and said, "How on Earth am I going to fall asleep at night without my glass of wine?"

I replied, "You're already tossing and turning throughout the night, so giving up that wine can only make things better."

She looked confused. "No, the wine helps me unwind and relaxes me. I haven't had a night in quite some time where I've tried to fall asleep without wine helping me with that."

That's when I told her, "Many people think alcohol helps them fall asleep, and yes, sometimes it does. The problem is that, more often than not, it interferes with the *quality* of your sleep. The tossing and turning? It's likely a result of the alcohol, and my bet is that giving it up will help you sleep better. It all goes back to that blood sugar balance that we've come back to over and over again throughout your coaching. Alcohol negatively affects your blood sugar levels. The interesting thing about alcohol is that everyone's body responds differently to it. For some people, blood sugar drops immediately after consuming alcohol, while in others, it spikes quickly, which is then followed by a precipitous drop. You know how it feels to crash in the middle of the day—sugar cravings, bad moods, trouble focusing, and headaches. Even if you don't feel those things in the middle of the night, you can bet it's still affecting you in similar ways. If you "crash" in the middle of the night, you're going to have trouble sleeping. However your body responds to alcohol, you're in for a ride on the blood sugar roller coaster every time you consume it. So when you toss and turn all night long, or wake up in the morning and don't feel rested, think about how the drinks you consumed the previous evening may have caused your blood sugar to crash in the middle of the night, resulting in restless sleep."

Of course, as we discussed in a previous chapter, lack of sleep is well documented as a promoter of inflammation and weight gain (and so is stress—hence the reason Lisa and I had spent quite a bit of time focusing on stress management). It's all connected. Remember: Less alcohol equals better sleep equals less inflammation equals easier weight loss.

Now, you can certainly make alcohol a part of your balanced life *if* you aren't wanting to lose weight. But alcohol is only going to bring you further from your weight loss goal, so you've got to lose the booze to lose the weight. Ultimately the choice is, of course, yours; you just need to be aware that it will take longer to reach your weight loss goals if you decide to keep consuming alcohol. It's up to you to determine if it's worth it to you or not. If you're like Lisa, and you've tried everything under the sun, and still haven't been able to get to the bottom of it, it might be worth it to give it up and see what happens.

I suggested that Lisa cut it out altogether—at least for the time being—to give her body a break from processing it. She wouldn't have it. She so looked forward to that evening ritual that she was simply unwilling to give it up—at least not yet.

Now, we all have different goals. I've learned that part of being a good coach is achieving a balance between tough love, and at the same time, meeting clients where they are, at that moment in time, with a caring, non-judgmental approach. At that point, I could say anything I wanted, but Lisa wasn't ready to give up the alcohol. Her goals weren't worth it to her to make that sacrifice, so instead we started with small steps. She said, "Tell me what I can do to just to make the wine less bad."

First, I encouraged her to try to drink as far away from bedtime as possible. She laughed when I told her to not take that the wrong way—I wasn't encouraging a morning Happy Hour! If she's going to drink a glass of wine, then it's best to have it earlier in the evening, and preferably with a meal. Since alcohol negatively affects blood sugars, balancing it with protein, fat, and carbohydrates (PFC) is crucial in order to keep those blood sugar levels as stable as possible. Then I told her that if she does have alcohol near bedtime, it's even more important to have a bedtime snack. Cheese and olives are a great, fat-filled, and healthy snack to keep you balanced, and their flavors pair well with wine. Lastly, I reminded her to have a big glass of water before bed, too, since alcohol can dehydrate the body.

Of course, not all drinks are created equal. I wasn't actually as concerned about Lisa's red wine—it's far less sugary than a lot of cocktail options out there. An easy rule of thumb is: the sweeter the wine, the higher in sugar it is.

When it comes to white or red, I say drink whichever you love. You may have heard that red wine has more antioxidant power than white, but to get in the amount of resveratrol that has been suggested to improve heart health, you would have to drink more than a few glasses (somewhere around 200!) to get that benefit. No way was I about to recommend that to Lisa, or anyone, so instead I recommended drinking a glass of whichever she likes best, while keeping in mind that the drier it is, the less sugar it has.

While Lisa was having wine most nights, she also confessed to me that on the weekends, her drink of choice was a Cosmopolitan. The problem with that is that many mixed and specialty drinks are high in sugar and/or artificial sweeteners...and who knows what else. From a nutritional standpoint, one of the biggest concerns with alcohol is not always the substance itself, but all the junk added to it. Unfortunately, to make matters worse, liquor isn't regulated like food, so manufacturers aren't required to list ingredients or even nutrition facts. Because of this, you can be sure that icky artificial flavorings, artificial sweeteners, colorings, preservatives, and other chemical ingredients are included in your favorite fancy drinks. I mean really, how can they *possibly* make vodka taste like "birthday cake" without using something artificial?!

In fact, I've come to believe that the dreaded hangover is more the result of the sugar and junk in the drinks rather than the booze. Of course, too much booze can certainly cause you to feel terrible the next day as your body tries to detoxify and recover from the damage, but more often than not, it seems like most hangovers can be prevented by choosing drinks that are less sugary and artificially sweetened (and balanced with plenty of fat on the side!).

Lisa was open to trying other drink options that might be able to bring her closer to her weight loss goal without completely giving up alcohol. So I gave her a few ideas to get started.

When it comes to alcohol, I think the gold standard is keeping it simple: vodka or tequila mixed with soda water and fresh squeezed lime…lots and lots of fresh squeezed lime (I'm talking a whole lime's-worth!). It's refreshing and free of added sugar and artificial sweeteners. Stick with clear spirits, like vodka, tequila, and gin, since liqueurs like amaretto, rum, and crème de Menthe have plenty of added sugar. I don't recommend beer since it is full of grains and carbs, both of which I recommend limiting, and no one wants a beer belly! Instead, I suggest hard cider as an alternative. Hard cider is a fermented alcoholic beverage made from fruit juice. It is important, however, to be careful of which cider you choose because the sugar content varies significantly depending on the brand. I recommend aiming for under 10 grams of sugar per 12-ounce serving. Some brands have 24 grams of sugar, which is almost equivalent to drinking a can of pop!

One of my favorite options I gave Lisa that's not as widely available at bars (yet!) is the kombucha cocktail. If you want to be the most popular person at a party, bring this cocktail! I actually made this drink as part of a TV show segment, and everyone loved the idea! Kombucha is a fizzy, fermented tea drink that's been getting a lot of attention lately. It's full of probiotics (beneficial bacteria), making it good for your gut, and therefore, your waistline. By itself, kombucha does contain a very small amount of alcohol, but it's such a trace amount that it likely won't affect you. Personally, I think even by itself, it tastes a lot like hard cider. I love that it hardly has any sugar, and instead, it's full of stuff that's GOOD for you!

Throwing a college party? Pour it into a wine glass and your friends probably won't even notice it's booze-less. If you don't want it to be booze-less, you can add a shot of vodka or tequila to your favorite flavor of kombucha to make a healthier mixed drink. Mixing with kombucha means you're simultaneously combating the damage from the alcohol as you drink it. A little oxymoronic, yes, but again, these tips are for you only if you aren't willing to give up alcohol completely. Of course, balancing that alcohol with a PFC meal or snack will ensure your blood sugar doesn't spike then take a nosedive.

Lo and behold, it didn't take Lisa long to not only give up her red wine, but to choose to *keep* it out. She was frustrated when she came into my office for her first appointment, but she had to get to the point where she was beyond frustrated before real change happened. Lisa was working her tail off at her job, in her household, and in multiple areas with me—especially that stress area of hers—yet, despite her hard effort, the pounds still weren't coming off as quickly as she wanted. Until she was really at her wit's end with the stubborn weight, she wasn't ready to say goodbye to her evening friend. That was okay—she had to come to that decision on her own, and sometimes it takes hitting a wall to get there. Lisa was onboard and it didn't take her long to reap the benefits of letting go of the wine—and that pesky, stubborn weight.

Fast forward to one month after Lisa put the cork in her wine consumption: "I'm ecstatic to be losing weight…but, I don't get it. It can't be the calories in the wine I've cut because I'm eating more calories than ever now and losing weight, yet no weight loss until saying "bye" to wine. What gives?"

I reminded Lisa that calories had nothing to do with it up to this point and recapped some of the reasons why it's wise to avoid alcohol altogether when weight loss is a goal. When you consume alcohol, burning off stored body fat is put on the back burner, while your liver first focuses on metabolizing and excreting the alcohol—which your body identifies as a toxin. You need your liver in tip-top shape to lose weight. Taking a break from booze allows your liver to focus on metabolizing fat and processing toxins, which will speed up your weight loss. This is key. It was also well worth reminding Lisa, as she experienced firsthand, how alcohol affects sleep. Alcohol was interfering with her ability to sleep soundly. Giving up the alcohol wasn't only giving her liver a break, but it was also allowing her hormones to get in balance during the night, which was critical for her to shed pounds. Sleep is that time to reset and recharge. For who knows how long, her body was never getting a break. On top of all that, she was stressed like no other, and routinely putting her body through stressful, restrictive diets that caused more stress and inflammation. No surprise she wasn't losing the weight!

If you're like Lisa and you are at your wit's end with your stubborn weight loss, you can baby step your way into not drinking alcohol like Lisa did, or you can lose those pounds faster by cutting it out altogether, which is my best recommendation. See what your body does when you aren't regularly ingesting something that it has to fight to get rid of. Take a break from the booze if you're serious about your weight loss goal. If giving up alcohol altogether seems like too great a challenge for you, I would still recommend doing a trial run, at least for a little while, to see how much it affects you. When you hit your goals, then absolutely have that celebratory drink! Just be sure not to "cheers" prematurely.

EPILOGUE

MOVING FORWARD

Whew. Take a deep breath. I realize that in the last eighteen chapters, I've given you *a lot* to digest (no pun intended)! Before I leave you, there are just a few more things that I want to share with you.

First, it's easier to understand and follow something when it's laid out, step-by-step, on a pretty page. That's why I created a guide for nearly every topic covered in this book! You can get all of those guides at dietitiancassie.com/bonus.

Second, I get it: you want results now. I understand you've been misguided and misled for far too long (I was, too). You're ready to shed those pounds once and for all. Now that I've given you valuable, life-changing, science-backed information, you've got the tools you need to finally get on the right track! I encourage you to be realistic with your expectations and patient with your body. We live in an instant, on-demand, drive-through, give-it-to-me-now society.

To get the results you want, you need to remember that quick fixes rarely lead to lasting results.

So, change your mindset and take advantage of the keys outlined in this book. This is your true process for healing and getting back in balance. You need to heal the damage done from restriction and deprivation. It took time for all that damage to build up. It will now take time for your body to trust that you are finally giving it what it needs to be the best body for you.

If you plateau after losing some weight, don't worry. This is normal. In fact, it's expected. If your body stays in a constant state of rapid change, it's too much of a shock. It needs time to figure out what the "new normal" is before it will move on to the next "new normal." When it happens, I implore you to stick with this program. Review some of the keys in this book, and see if there is an element that you've overlooked and can weave into your routine. If you have lots of inflammation, aren't sleeping, have a hormone problem, are stressed out, have a food sensitivity, or are dealing with one or more of the other factors I outlined for you, then your body is likely more focused on taking care of those issues than burning stored fat right now. Be patient and consistent while doing the things I've taught you, and your body will thank you by shedding pounds after it heals and finds balance.

There is one element that isn't outlined in this book, but it has been a groundbreaking factor for our clients. It is guided accountability for those times when you get stuck. Think of it this way: Do you know how celebrities stay fit? The answer is that they have a whole *team* of people who help them—a lot.

Right now, you have the information you need; you absolutely can take this journey on your own.

However, if you've found yourself in a place like the clients I've described in this book, and you're interested in having your very own personal team, you don't have to do this alone! We love helping clients accelerate their weight loss journey. When they run into roadblocks, we can quickly find solutions to their specific problems. Finding root causes and healing from the inside out is our specialty and joy. To learn more about our approach and what we can do for you, visit healthysimplelife.com.

Last but certainly not least, having a "why" matters. What's your motivation? Coming up with reasons why you want to accomplish a goal can make all the difference when you're facing challenging times. Sure, weight loss is a goal because it's nice to lose weight, but why do you really want to lose the weight? Is it because the extra pounds are affecting your joints and you want to be able to move without pain? Is your goal to travel freely when you get older, and it's too hard to move around as it is right now? Do you want to be able to play with your kids or grandkids, and not sit on the sidelines as you watch them grow up? Maybe your real motivation is to feel happy and comfortable in your own skin so that you can feel more confident and have better relationships. Write down the *real* reasons behind your specific goals and refer to them whenever you feel a dip in your motivation. This is worth it, because you are worth it.

What you do with this information is up to you! Remember, you can head over to dietitiancassie.com/bonus to find all of the in-depth guides from this book. The keys to unlocking your stubborn weight loss are right in front of you. Now, it's time to put them in the locks and start turning them!

ACKNOWLEDGEMENTS

Thank you to my friends and colleagues for reviewing the book. Your insight and suggestions have made this one of the reasons why I'm so proud to have it in the hands of the many readers who have struggled with weight loss. Thank you so much for offering encouragement, love, and support along the way.

Thanks to my amazing team at Healthy Simple Life® for holding down the fort while I had my head and heart very much in this book.

My deepest gratitude goes out to you, the reader, for giving me the opportunity to share the knowledge and insight I've gained from my own health journey and years of working with clients.

I am forever thankful that this book found its way into your hands and my hope and prayer is that you now apply the information so that it can transform your life.

It breaks my heart knowing there are so many others out there still suffering because of wrong health and weight loss advice. Too many people still feel like failures, like it's all their fault, like there's something wrong with them. If I could ask one thing of you, it would be this: Will you pay it forward? I'm sure there's a friend, family member, or coworker who could benefit from this information just as much as you will. Thank you in advance for joining me in the movement of un-brainwashing ourselves from conventional, flat-out wrong weight loss "wisdom" and spreading the truth so that we can be freed of dieting...forever.

RESOURCES

Recommended Supplements
Real Food Vitamins: www.rfvitamins.com

Book Guides
Available at www.dietitiancassie.com/bonus

Community Group and Daily Support
PFC Club Membership Program:
www.dietitiancassie.com/community

Want to bring Dietitian Cassie in as your next guest speaker?
Visit www.dietitiancassie.com/speaking/ to learn why she'll make for the perfect speaker at your next event.

Interested in personalized Nutrition and Lifestyle Coaching from Cassie and her team?
Visit www.dietitiancassie.com/coaching for information and to get started!

ABOUT THE AUTHOR

DIETITIAN CASSIE is leading a nutrition revolution. As a Registered, Licensed Dietitian, founder and CEO of the wellness company Healthy Simple Life®, and #1 International Best Selling Author, Dietitian Cassie has built a following of loyal fans by helping people with the root causes of their health issues—especially ones that healthcare practitioners often overlook. From major corporate events to personal client coaching, Cassie reveals the transformational power of real food and evidence-based nutrition to help people find freedom from diets and chronic health conditions.

Virtually every major media outlet—including CBS, ABC, WCCO, FOX News, Twin Cities Live television, CNN, TIME, Parade, Cosmopolitan, Self, and The Huffington Post—has covered Cassie's quest to debunk the lies and spread the truth about the food we eat.

When she's not speaking or working one-on-one with her clients, you can find her paddleboarding, running, rollerblading or biking around her favorite chain of lakes where she resides in Minneapolis, Minnesota.

A Personal Note from Dietitian Cassie:

Life's a journey, and I continually share the findings of my research and work with clients through exclusive emails delivered right to your inbox and my blog. I invite you to join me over at dietitiancassie.com.

Made in the USA
Middletown, DE
10 November 2016